To all my patients who have taught me so much and have been the real encouragement to write this book

To all my friends who supported me whilst I was putting this book together

To my friend and research assistant, Mr Jonathan Sims, whose help made this book possible

and

To Susan, Talita and Jemima for your constant inspiration, support, and love

Free From Pain

Principles of Lifestyle Medicine to help with musculoskeletal pain and arthritis. Advice from a Consultant Orthopaedic Surgeon.

Dr George Ampat
Consultant Orthopaedic Surgeon

Dr George Ampat FRCS works as a Consultant Orthopaedic Surgeon in the UK. After 30 years of a busy surgical practice, Dr. Ampat now aims to help patients with musculoskeletal pain with lifestyle changes, exercises, and diet rather than resorting to surgery.

DISCLAIMER – PLEASE READ THIS PRIOR TO USING THIS BOOK

Please note that the content of this book is for information only. The information provided is done so with the aim to enlighten readers and offer an alternative point of view about certain aspects of health which may not be well-known. The content is not intended to be a substitute for professional medical advice, diagnosis or treatment. Always seek the advice of your doctor or other qualified health provider with any questions you may have regarding a medical condition. Never disregard professional medical advice or delay seeking it because of something you have read in this book. If you think you may have a medical emergency, call your doctor, go to the nearest hospital emergency department, or call the emergency services immediately. If you choose to rely on any information provided in this book, you do so solely at your own risk.

Talita Cumi Ltd
681, Liverpool Road, Southport PR8 3NS
www.ampat.co.uk
www.freefrompain.org.uk

Printed in the United Kingdom

Ampat, George
Free From Pain - Principles of Lifestyle Medicine to help with musculoskeletaleletal pain and arthritis. Advice from a Consultant Orthopaedic Surgeon.
ISBN 978-0-9956769-5-4

Contents

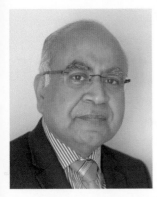

As a Consultant Orthopaedic Surgeon, it seemed easy for me to recommend injections or surgical interventions (operations) for patients with pain. It is a wonderful, if not an exhilarating experience when the surgery proceeds without any adverse events and the patient is satisfied with the outcome. When it all goes well, it seems like magic.

Sometimes, the magic does not happen. Occasionally, patients do not achieve the desired outcome from surgery. The patient may continue to experience the same pain even following their operation. Additionally, surgery may cause catastrophic results due to complications. When this happens, the patient is left with more problems following surgery than before.

When surgery has caused complications or when the desired results have not been achieved, the intervention cannot be undone. Patients may require further surgical interventions, like removal of the implant or revision of the procedure. Though it is possible to remove an implant, the patient cannot be returned to their pre-surgical state of health. Other patients may need more medications to control the pain, which they have to consume for the rest of their life. Patients have to live with the effects of the operation, whether they like them or not.

All surgeons and other health professionals are fully aware of this and are very conscientious when recommending surgery for their patients. In many countries, registries exist for certain surgical procedures. In the United Kingdom, the National Joint Registry monitors the outcome of all joint replacements. Evidence from these registries has provided further insight into the long-term results of surgery, using data from the entire population. Whilst research publications may only be from select centres of excellence, results of registries are from all centres and provide the population mean of any intervention. With all this newfound evidence, it has become apparent that many patients do not actually require injections or operations. They may just need lifestyle medicine advice.

Lifestyle medicine is not a single intervention or procedure that will provide relief from pain or control arthritis. Lifestyle medicine is a collection of multiple small measures that, when collectively performed, provides improvement.

Unfortunately, there isn't a book which clearly explains and provides evidence based lifestyle measures that could be useful to patients with musculoskeletal pain. In that endeavour, I have created this book. This book provides 15 areas of lifestyle medicine that would be useful to help with arthritis and pain. In isolation, none of these measures will provide the magic cure. However, the collective use of these methods will provide the tools to optimise health and decrease pain. The book is also likely to help patients who may not be experiencing any arthritic pain but who may just desire to adopt a better lifestyle to improve their musculoskeletal and general health.

I would like to make it clear that surgery is by no means bad, and it can be good when performed for the right reasons. However, there is an excessive dependence on surgery and injections.

The guide has been created to provide concise, evidence-based advice regarding non-operative approaches to musculoskeletal pain. It supplies educational information about what I believe to be the most important pillars of a healthy lifestyle. For instance, various aspects of lifestyle medicine, including diet, exercise and sleep, are discussed throughout the book. For each aspect, findings from research studies are presented to showcase how they can optimise health and quality of life. The guide also provides citations of the referenced studies, allowing further reading and reflection opportunities. The book is intended to enable patients to independently read about the changes they can make to their lifestyle in order to reduce the threat of disability and ill-health. As a result of the advice provided, patients may have a second chance to reclaim their health and take active steps to a pain-free, happy, and energetic lifestyle.

Action to improve health is more vital now than ever. With our ever-ageing population and our increasing life expectancy, we all need to make changes to increase the quality of our later years. We may now live 10, or even 20, years longer than people did many years ago. Let us ensure that these extra years of life are filled with happiness and energy and are pain-free.

Additional information

We also have an exercise book available – the *"Free From Pain Exercise Book"*. This exercise book contains evidence-based material and health-related stories highlighting why exercise can be so beneficial for health. I hope that the information inspires readers to engage in more physical activity. The exercise book also contains exercises designed to improve balance and mobility in older adults whilst reducing musculoskeletal pain. These exercises have been compiled into a 12-week functional rehabilitation programme, which can be done independently at home.

If you would like to purchase the *"Free From Pain Exercise Book"*, it is available separately at Amazon or at www.freefrompain.org.uk.

If you are interested in the *"Free From Pain"* exercises, you can view them on our YouTube channel: www.youtube.com/c/GeorgeAmpat The *"Free From Pain"* playlist in this channel provides all the videos of the exercises.

I wish to thank my research team for their numerous hours of hard work in researching, compiling, editing, formatting and repeating the process over and over again till we reached a final product. Without them this book would not have been possible.

I sincerely hope you enjoy this book.

Dr George Ampat

Dr Ampat's research team

Mr. Jonathan Sims, BSc

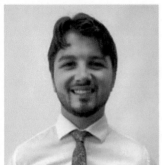

A Lancaster University graduate with a degree in psychology, Mr. Sims now works as Dr Ampat's research assistant. In his spare time he enjoys travelling and reading.

Dr. Jemima George, MBBS

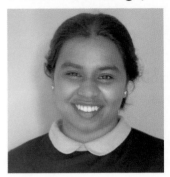

Dr George works as a junior doctor in the North East of England. In her free time she enjoys working with young children as part of church and playing the piano.

FREE FROM PAIN is an acronym and incorporates the main pillars of Lifestyle Medicine

Fear

Reduction

Exercise

Early with

Food from plants

Rest and relaxation

Organisation (family & friends)

Motivation (ikigai) to decrease

Pain from

Arthritis and to

Increase

Natural strength

Chapter 1 – Blue Zones

Introduction

We are fortunate to exist in a modern society where, in recent times, the quality of healthcare and hygiene has improved greatly throughout the world. These developments have allowed for the global average life expectancy to rise steadily over the last century. Nowhere is this more evident than in the UK. We have one of the best medical care systems in the world. We are pioneers in the field of medical research and world leaders in the development of healthcare technology. Despite this, we struggle with issues of obesity and the pressures of an ageing population. While it is true that we now live longer, later-life disability remains a significant problem. In other words, leading a long life does not correlate with leading one *"Free From Pain"*.

Blue Zones – what are they?

There are places where this isn't the situation – where the population leads fulfilling lives, free from health problems and disability. In some parts of the world, people live longer and with fewer health problems than anywhere else on Earth. These places are collectively known as "Blue Zones". In his book "The Secrets of a Long Life", Dan Buettner highlighted the "Blue Zones". He identified five areas: Okinawa (Japan); Sardinia (Italy); Nicoya (Costa Rica); Icaria (Greece) and Loma Linda (California). These areas hold values and ideologies that enable their residents to live long and well. As a result, nowhere else has more centenarians (people who live 100+ years) than these places [1].

The Okinawa experience

What are the differences between our nation and these Blue Zones? Why do the

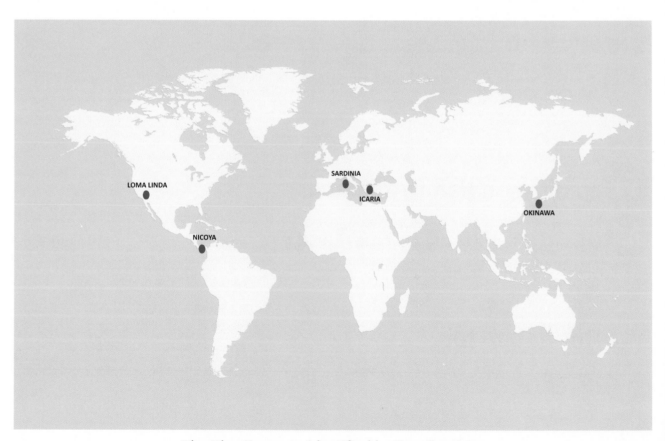

The Blue Zones as identified by Dan Buettner

people of the UK face the prospect of later-life illness and disability whilst those in these Blue Zones do not? Contrary to what one might expect, Blue Zones are typically neither wealthy nor medically advanced. Okinawa, one of the Blue Zones, is actually the poorest province in Japan. However, the people here are rich in their sense of community, family, and friends [2]. They form social support networks called "maois". This small friendship network created at a young age meets every day to have a chat and a drink. If one member does not turn up, the other four go and find the fifth to check up on them. The Okinawans also restrict their calorie intake by following the age-old mantra of "Hara Hachi Bu". This term translates to "eat until you are 80% full." [1]

The Loma Linda experience
Excellent health is not just the privilege of the residents of a remote Japanese island: Blue Zones are also seen in the western world. For instance, circumstances are very similar in another Blue Zone – Loma Linda, California – where a Seventh-Day Adventist Church is established. The Seventh-Day Adventist Church is a protestant organisation with many locations worldwide, but there is a concentration of Seventh-Day Adventists in Loma Linda. The Seventh-Day Adventist Church is known for presenting a "health message", emphasising diet and lifestyle as important factors. Like in Okinawa, the sense of community here is strong, and Church members are encouraged to volunteer in their local neighbourhood. Adventists also observe the Sabbath on Saturdays [1]. During these 24 hours, they focus on family, camaraderie, and spending time with like-minded friends. This allows Adventists to appreciate the closeness of their relationships, resulting in good mental health.

Mental health in the UK vs. Blue Zones
Whilst the overall mental health of the population in the Blue Zones is good, here in the UK, it is a different story. In the UK, one in four people experience a mental health problem every year [3]. This is a chief concern as it is now established that poor mental health can be detrimental to physical health. One study found that mental illness can decrease life expectancy more than the effects of heavy smoking and suggested that recurrent depression can reduce life expectancy by 11 years [4]. The sense of companionship and lack of loneliness felt in the Blue Zones by the elderly prevents them from experiencing such adverse effects, enabling them to live longer and happier lives.

Advantages of a predominantly plant-based diet
Currently, diet is a common topic clouded by contradictory expert advice and countless dietary variations. With so many diverse recommendations, it is difficult to know which diet is best. However, one factor of diet has been emphasized repeatedly– the need for more minimally processed or unprocessed plant-based foods. Processed food is food that has undergone any form of processing. Processing can range from washing to industrial cooking. Industrial cooking combines food with numerous unhealthy additives to increase flavour and shelf life. On the contrary, fresh vegetables cooked at home do not contain these additives, which is a good choice for better health.

Such fresh and organic vegetables enrich the Okinawan diet. The citizens in Okinawa eat over 300 grams of vegetables daily in a diet low in calories and carbohydrates [2]. As a result, most residents maintain a body mass index of 18–22 throughout their lives [2]. Furthermore, studies have found that elders in the Okinawan community have low cholesterol levels and impressively clean arteries, reducing their risk of cardiovascular disease by an astonishing 80% [2]. On the other hand, cardiovascular disease (CVD) is a significant problem in the UK, causing over a quarter of the overall deaths in the country [5].

Cancer in the UK vs Blue Zones

Along with cardiovascular disease, cancer is a massive burden on our society and an enormous concern for us all. In 2016, there were 1.8 million people diagnosed with cancer in England [6]. It may be easy to assume that little can be done to prevent the disease. However, a study on Adventists shows otherwise. Adventists are encouraged to adopt a vegetarian/vegan lifestyle with a diet high in peas, beans, and nuts. The study showed that vegetarian Adventists reduced the risk of bowel cancer by 23% and prostate cancer by 35% compared to non-vegetarian Adventists [7].

Exercise the Blue Zone way – No hi-tech gyms but moderate activity throughout the day.

As a country, our obsession with gyms and weight-loss programmes is unparalleled. Whilst we search for quick-fix solutions to lose weight, the Okinawan people incorporate physical activity into their daily lives – no personal trainers or gyms are needed. Exercise becomes a part of everyday life and gives Okinawans a purpose. As a result, many Okinawan elders run and manage organic vegetable gardens and sell the excess produce well into their 90s and 100s. The majority also grow up practising karate, kendo, or dancing [2]. These forms of physical activity are goal-orientated for reasons other than weight loss and there is a consistent, positive attitude toward staying active throughout their entire life. This "little and often" approach to exercise helps the Okinawans maintain their health by incorporating activity into daily life.

What can be done?

The ideologies and diets adopted by the people of Blue Zones have had a remarkable effect on their health, happiness, and life expectancy. Here in the UK, we can embrace the lifestyle measures of these fantastic places to reduce the levels of disability and adverse health conditions. Dan Buettner recommends the "Power 9" formula as follows [1]:

1. Move naturally. Instead of visiting the gym, walk to and from work, shops, and schools.
2. Have a purpose – "ikigai". The day should be filled with activity, either for the family or the community.
3. Decrease your stress. Take an afternoon nap, pray, or meditate regularly.
4. "Hara hachi bu" – do not fill your tummy. Stop when the tummy is 80% full.
5. Follow a plant-based diet. Limit meats to a small portion once a week.

6. Have a glass of wine daily, but do not binge over the weekend.
7. Be part of a social group.
8. Love and serve your family.
9. Join a network of friends. Happiness is contagious.

Chapter 2 – Avoid Sedentary lifestyle

Introduction

Sedentary behaviour involves very low energy expenditure. This behaviour includes sitting at a desk, reclining, relaxing in front of a television or lying down. Although it may not apply to everyone, a good proportion of society leads to sedentary lifestyles. This is especially true for older adults and individuals who may have retired. A study published in 2015 explored the length of time adults over 60 are sedentary during their waking day [1]. The study revealed that, on average, adults over 60 are inactive for 9.4 hours of their waking day. This value equates to around 65% to 80% of their day [1]. One reason is that sitting and watching TV for long hours is very common among the elderly, contributing to inactivity. In addition, social isolation, which is common in older people, can also contribute to increased sedentary behaviour and reduced physical activity [2].

Harm from sedentary behaviour

Spending up to 65% to 80% of a waking day inactive can significantly impact the well-being of an individual, potentially causing many adverse effects on a person's mental and physical health. Unfortunately, inactivity contributes to the causation of chronic diseases and results in significant reductions in quality of life and longevity [3]. A few conditions that are associated with inactivity include:

1. Type II diabetes
2. Metabolic syndrome (a combination of diabetes, high blood pressure and obesity)
3. Coronary heart disease
4. Stroke
5. Dementia
6. Cancers (colon, breast and endometrial)

Sarcopenia

Loss of muscle mass is termed sarcopenia. Sarcopenia may be a silent killer in the elderly, and being sedentary increases the loss of muscle mass (sarcopenia) [3]. A

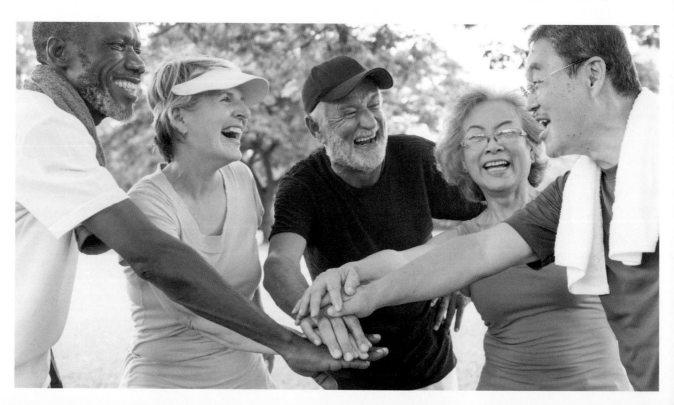

decrease in muscle mass causes balance issues which can lead to an increased risk of falls. Falls may result in fractures such as a broken hip. This may then require surgery to fix or replace the hip. Recovery following the surgery is also prolonged when muscle mass is decreased. The good news, however, is that sarcopenia is not an unavoidable consequence of ageing. Being active and avoiding sedentary behaviour can rectify the condition.

Mental health issues and dementia

Physical inactivity can also cause mental health problems, including depression. In fact, up to one-third of depression is caused by inactivity [3]. On the contrary, being physically active can prevent 20 to 30% of depression [3]. Sedentary behaviour also leads to an enlarged threat of dementia. Yan and the team reviewed relevant previous studies and concluded that, based on the evidence available, sedentary behaviour was significantly associated with an increased risk of developing dementia [4].

Self-reported quality of life

Health-related quality of life refers to perceived health or well-being [5]. In other words, it is how individuals perceive their own physical and mental health. Kim and Lee's 2019 study involved 1,415 adults over the age of 65. The participants were asked to report how long they sat down and were sedentary each day. They were also asked to report how they perceived their own health. The results of the study showed that participants who reported longer sitting times were more likely to report lower quality of self-perceived health, while those who reported shorter sitting times self-reported higher quality of

health [5]. Interestingly, this relationship was stronger for people over 75 years old than for participants 75 years or under [5].

Death from any cause

"All-cause mortality" and "Systemic reviews" are terms commonly used in research. "All-cause mortality" denotes death from any cause. "Systematic review" involves research combining the results of many studies on the same subject. De Rezende and colleagues conducted a systematic review to investigate the impact of sedentary behaviour on various health conditions in older adults over 60 years of age. Their review found that greater sedentary time was associated with an increased risk of all-cause mortality in older adults and that inactivity resulted in obesity, increased waist circumference, and metabolic syndrome [6].

Physical activity and cancer

Even cancer can be caused by decreased physical activity. Conversely, routine physical activity has been found to reduce the incidence of cancers. A study by Lugo and team reviewed the literature available and, based on the results, concluded that physical activity reduced the risk of colon, breast, lung and endometrial cancers [7]. In addition to preventing cancers, physical activity was also shown to increase survival following cancer diagnosis and decrease both cancer and all-cause mortality rates [7]. Physical activity can also improve functional status and quality of life during chemotherapy and treatment for cancer in patients who have been diagnosed [7].

Compression of morbidity: checking out of "Hotel Earth."

Life expectancy has increased massively in

the last 100 years. Life expectancy was in the 60s in the 1920s but had risen to the 80s by 2020. However, does a longer life expectancy translate to a longer and healthier life, or does it mean a more extended period of disability and suffering? Humans are programmed to die eventually; hence, ensuring good quality of life before death is as crucial as increasing life expectancy.

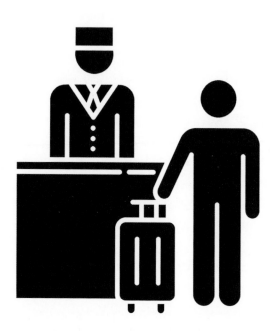

As human beings, we check into "Hotel Earth" when we are born. At some point, we have to check out of "Hotel Earth". This checkout process is crucial. The checkout can be short and sweet after a beautiful stay, or the checkout could be prolonged and painful. While most humans go through a period of chronic illness before death, attempts must be made to shorten this period as much as possible. Decreasing the period of chronic disease before death is termed "compression of morbidity". Doing so, and living a long and fruitful life with only a very short period of chronic illness and incapacity before death is the dream ticket to hope for. Fortunately,

numerous health strategies can aid in the compression of morbidity. The most effective and single primary intervention, which reduces the threat of chronic conditions developing, is exercise [8].

The Runners' Study – can exercise damage me and my joints?

"The Runners' Study" began in 1984 and sought to investigate the effects of exercise on health and disability [9]. The investigation covered 21 years and compared the later life disabilities of 538 runners with 423 healthy non-runners. Participants were all over the age of 50 at the onset of the study in 1984. Throughout the study, disability was always less in the runners, and runners took 12 years longer to reach the same level of disability as non-runners (19 years vs. seven years) [9]. The worry and anxiety of every exercise enthusiast is that the increased exercise would cause the joints to wear out. This study, however, proved otherwise - with runners having fewer knee and hip replacements [9]. Moreover, time to death was postponed by eight years for the runners. The increased life expectancy was double in runners compared to those who did not run (16 years vs. eight years) [9]. At the 19-year point of the study, only 15% of runners had passed away, whilst 34% of non-runners had died [9]. The findings of this study show how moderately strenuous exercise can postpone disability even further than it postpones death. Therefore, as a result of exercising, people can extend their lifespan and reduce the number of years spent with disability.

What can be done?
The effects of a sedentary lifestyle can be universally damaging. Even though many

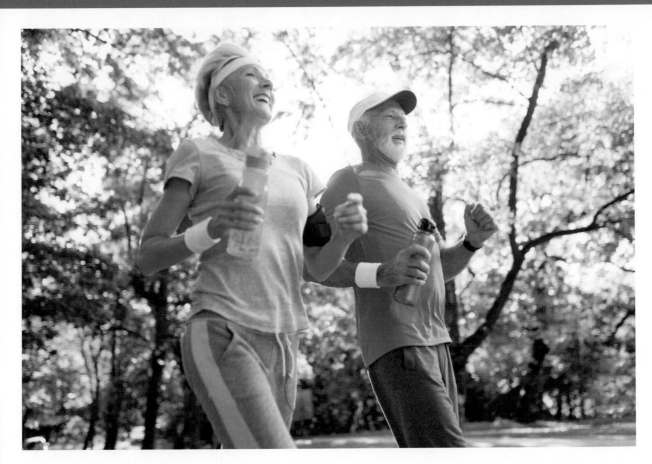

recent advances in health care and medicine have increased life expectancy, getting older still increases the likelihood of illness. This risk is further increased by the sedentary lifestyle many older adults live. Therefore, measures must be taken to tackle the ever-increasing levels of inactivity, particularly in older adults. Simple, minor lifestyle changes can equate to a higher quality of life. Crucially, increased activity benefits the individual and can reduce social and financial costs to society. So, let us move more and let us age healthily.

Thankfully, time spent being sedentary can be easily reduced. The National Health Service in the United Kingdom recommends that people over the age of 65, who are generally fit and well, should aim to do 150 minutes of moderate physical activity per week. This includes walking and leisure cycling [10]. Moderate physical activity is defined as activity that would make a person slightly breathless. The breathlessness during moderate physical activity is mild and will prevent a person from singing while performing the activity, but it will not prevent the person from talking. In contrast, during vigorous physical activity, one cannot sing or talk continuously without stopping and taking a breath. Similarly, if you can sing while performing an activity, the activity is mild physical activity and cannot be classed as a moderately strenuous physical activity.

Everyday activities such as carrying groceries and gardening with tools can also make a big difference, as they aid in strengthening muscles and protecting joints. Physical activity should not be considered a chore. In addition, it is not necessary to join a gymnasium and lift heavy weights. Physical activity should be merely incorporated into daily life, with

individuals getting some form of exercise
as they cruise through the day. Walking to
and from work, the shops or the post office
are examples that can be followed easily.

It is important to find the balance between
exercising to improve your health and
pushing yourself too much, which can
cause lasting damage itself. If you have any
questions about what exercise is suitable,
please go and talk to a healthcare
professional as they will be able to advise
you personally.

Chapter 3 – Under-Standing Over-Sitting

Introduction

Before the industrial revolution, people only sat an average of 5 hours per day [1]. As civilisations have developed, humans have become increasingly accustomed to spending a significant amount of their waking day sitting down. Now, 25% of people from developed countries sit for eight or more hours per day [2]. This equates to around half of the time that they are awake. Older adults (65 years or older) spend an even longer time sitting down; some individuals may spend as much as 15 hours a day sitting [1]. Nowadays, we can even find a life partner while sitting down and browsing online. Gone are the days when dancing was required for dating.

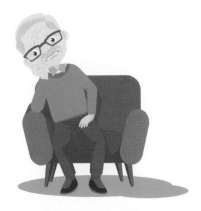

In developed countries, 25% of people sit for eight or more hours a day

This increase in over-sitting is because modern environments are created to foster and encourage the behaviour. Some of the most common sedentary activities include sitting at work all day, travelling to work, and sitting in a domestic setting (e.g. at home). Consequently, sitting has become an important research topic and is now linked to reduced life expectancy, poor health, and frailty.

Life expectancy

The impact that excessive sitting can have on our physical health has received more academic and public attention in the past decade. Research carried out by Chau and team reviewed six studies that had investigated the effects of sitting on health [2]. The six studies contained data from 595,086 adults. Daily total sitting time was assessed and followed for an average of 2.8 years. Chau and colleagues concluded that each hour spent sitting daily was associated with a 2% increase in the risk of death [2]. The study also identified that this risk increased further for those adults who sit for more than seven hours a day [2]. Adults who sit for ten hours a day were estimated to have a 34% increased risk of dying [2]. Therefore, we need to consider how much of our day is spent sitting and how this could impact our life expectancy.

Smoking has been identified as one of the greatest public health disasters of the 20th century. With that in mind, it is worrying to know that some research studies have suggested that sitting is the modern-day equivalent of smoking. Research carried out by Veerman and team found that smoking a single cigarette reduces your life expectancy by around 11 minutes [3].

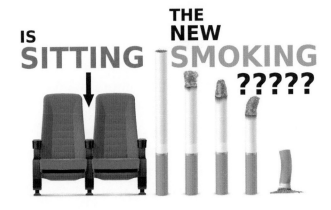

Their study also identified that for those over the age of 25, sitting for an hour daily reduced life expectancy by 11 minutes [3]. This shows that daily sitting should be just as much of a health concern as smoking, indicating just how damaging excessive sitting can be to health and life expectancy.

Chronic Illnesses

Spending prolonged periods of the day sitting may have repercussions on life expectancy, quality of life, and overall health. Gomez-Cabello and team investigated the influence of sitting on body composition in 457 women. In these women, active behaviour was defined as walking for more than one hour daily. Sedentary behaviour was defined as sitting for more than four hours a day [4]. The researchers found that women who sat for more than four hours a day had higher weight, BMI, waist circumference and fat mass than those who sat less [4]. These results reveal that sitting for prolonged periods vastly increases the risk of being overweight or obese.

As many as 35 chronic conditions and diseases are associated with sedentary behaviour. Research carried out by Levine and team identified that many of the modern health concerns the world faces today, such as obesity, cardiovascular disease, various forms of cancer and Type II diabetes, can be attributed to excessive sitting [1]. This is supported by the literature, where sitting for more than eight hours a day has been shown to increase the risk of dying of cancer by 15% and the threat of developing cardiovascular disease by 14% [5]. The dangers of sitting for such excessive periods can be so severe that it also doubles the risk of developing

Type II diabetes [5]. These conditions reduce the quality of life and can shorten life expectancy. Sitting for prolonged periods has also been found to increase the risk of developing depression by nearly 14% [5].

Neck and back pain

Sitting for long periods can also have a considerable negative effect on our musculoskeletal health. There is a direct link between sitting for long periods and developing neck and lower back pain.

The association between sitting and lower back pain was investigated by Gupta and team. 201 blue-collar workers were required to wear devices that measured their sitting time for four consecutive working days. They were also asked to report the intensity of their lower back pain in the previous month. The results showed a significant association between higher total sitting time, whether at work or leisure time, and increased intensity of lower back pain [7].

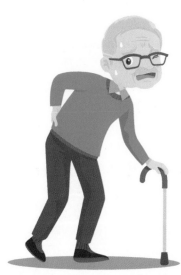

Sitting for long periods can have a negative impact on our musculoskeletal health

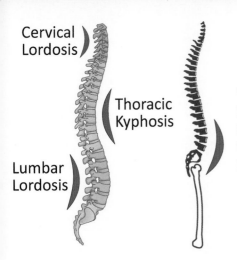

When standing the inward curve (lumbar lordosis) of the lower back is maintained.

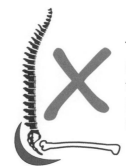

The inward curve (lumbar lordosis) of the lower back is lost when seated at 90 degrees

The spine has a natural forward curve in the lower back (lumbar lordosis), as shown in the image on the left. This curve is maintained when standing but is lost when seated on a horizontal, flat seat at 90 degrees

Sitting and its effects on the anatomy of the spine

Sitting in a flat seat causes lower back pain because it alters the natural anatomy of the spine. The spine is not completely straight. If looked at from the side, it has a natural double "S" shaped curve. In the neck and lower back, the spine curves forwards toward the centre of the body. This inwards curve is called lordosis and is referred to as cervical lordosis in the neck and lumbar lordosis in the lower back. The backwards component of the curve is where the spine bends away from the centre of the body. The backwards bend is called kyphosis. This is found behind the chest wall in the thoracic spine and in the bottom of the spine at the pelvis. The bend behind the rib cage is called thoracic kyphosis, and the bend in the pelvis is called sacral kyphosis. The alternating forward and backward curves increase stability. It is essential that these curves are maintained, as this keeps the discs in a functional position. Sitting in a flat or a horizontal seat reduces the backward curve in the lower back region.

Decreasing the backward curve in the lower back is called 'reduction of lumbar lordosis'. A decrease in lumbar lordosis increases the pressure on the intervertebral discs of the lower back and is associated with lower back pain [6]. To maintain lumbar lordosis, the hips should be a few inches higher than the knees when sitting down. Many chairs have flat seats, which alter lumbar lordosis, potentially contributing to lower back pain. Hence, it is recommended that we sit on seats that are sloped downwards to maintain lumbar lordosis.

Sitting and its effects on the intervertebral discs of the lower back

The discs in the spine are plump and cushion the vertebral bones, keeping them apart. If cut into, the discs are similar to a jam doughnut. The dough-like outer covering of the disc is called the "annulus fibrosus", and the jam-like inside is called the "nucleus pulposus". Under the increased pressure caused by sitting, the disc may become compressed at the front, squeezing the jam-like centre (nucleus pulposus) towards the rear [6]. As more of

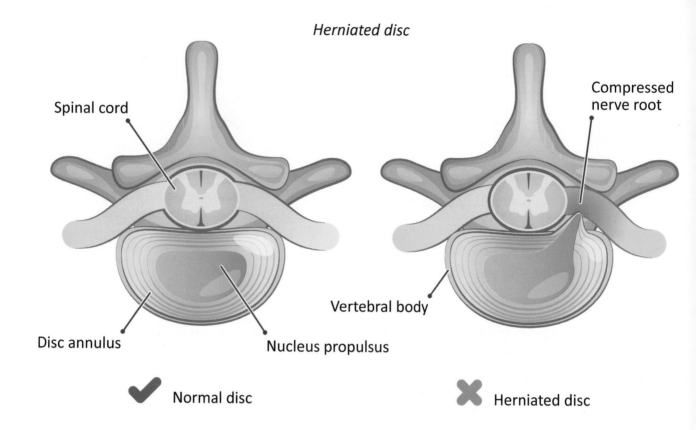

Herniated disc

Spinal cord

Compressed nerve root

Disc annulus

Nucleus propulsus

Vertebral body

✔ Normal disc

✖ Herniated disc

the jam-like content is pushed into the rear of the disc, the disc casing becomes stretched. If the disc cracks under the pressure, the jam-like contents will leak out, potentially causing compression of the spinal cord or nerve roots going into the legs in what is known as a disc herniation [6]. This can cause leg pain (sciatica) which can be extremely painful and debilitating and may be worse than the back pain itself.

A classic paper released in 1966 by Nachemson calculated the actual pressure applied to the lumbar discs when the body is in different positions, including when seated. He found that if a person weighing 70 kilograms is standing, their third lumbar disc (L3) is under around 100 kilograms of pressure [8]. When seated in an unsupported upright position, this pressure increases to 142 kilograms, a rise of 42% [8]. Furthermore, sitting and tilting forward

20 degrees, which many office workers may be guilty of when working at desks, further increases this pressure to around 191 kilograms, almost double the load when standing [8]. These results show that sitting, and especially on flat and horizontal seats, increases the stress applied to the discs of the lower back, enlarging the risk of degeneration and disc prolapse.

How to sit
It is, therefore, important to sit in a position that is supportive to the spine. Ideally the angle of the thigh in relation to the torso should be approximately 135 degrees when seated. In 1953, Dr Jay J Keegan repeatedly X-rayed the lower back of four healthy volunteers. Each x-ray was taken in a different position. Dr Keegan identified that lumbar lordosis was dependent on the trunk-thigh angle. When the trunk-thigh angle is 90 degrees, which

is often the case when sitting in regular chairs, lumbar lordosis is lost. However, when the trunk thigh angle is increased to 135 degrees, lumbar lordosis is restored [9].

Sitting prevents the maintenance of the intervertebral discs

Another aspect to consider regarding sitting and its effects on back pain is the mechanisms behind how the intervertebral discs receive their nutrients. The discs do not have a direct blood supply as the blood vessels only reach up to the edge of the bone. The discs obtain oxygen, water and nutrients only through diffusion from the ends of the bone. Such diffusion and passage of nutrients in enhanced by movement. This is akin to how the eyes are kept hydrated. Automatic and subconscious blinking is an evolutionary adaptation which ensures that the cornea (the front of the eye) remains moist and functional. If the eyes were to stay open for too long, they would dry and could potentially cause blindness. Blinking lubricates the eyes by spreading tears across the surface, ensuring they remain undamaged. Similarly, movement allows the intervertebral discs to absorb nutrients and disperse waste products. Cyclical loading of the discs with walking and mild jogging causes the discs to repeatedly compress and decompress under the weight of the body with each step. The discs then act like a sponge, pushing out waste material while soaking up nutrients and water. This mechanism is called "fluid pumping". The process significantly increases the transportation of molecules into and out of the disc, including enzymes and hormones essential in keeping the discs healthy [10]. In the eye, there are warning mechanisms that force us to blink if the eyes become dry. Unfortunately, such warning mechanisms do not exist in the lower back. Thus, a lack of movement from excessive sitting may disrupt the transfer of vital nutrients into and out of the disc, contributing to disc degeneration and consequent back pain [10]. Hence, sitting in one position without movement can contribute to disc degeneration and low back pain by simply preventing the "fluid pumping" process.

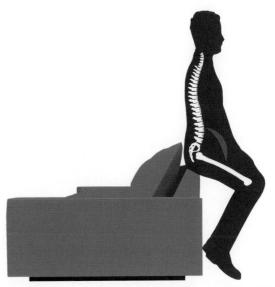

Perching on the back of your sofa will maintain an appropriate trunk-thigh angle, preserving lumbar lordosis

What can you do?

Due to the dangers of prolonged sitting, it is important to stand and move at constant intervals. Another option would be to sit with the hips higher than the knees. Saddle chairs allow this. Sitting on a regular sofa decreases lumbar lordosis, but perching on the back of the sofa can restore lumbar lordosis. In addition, this position forces one to stand and change position constantly. This allows movement to occur between the discs and the vertebrae.

Chapter 4 – Television and Its Effects on Brain Function

Introduction

Television viewing is on the increase. In 2020, around 27 million households in the UK owned a TV. This is nearly 95% of all households in the country [1]. Consequently, it is no surprise that watching TV is a common daily activity and is regarded as a mainstream cultural pastime. For many, it is a window to the rest of the world and the primary source of news and education. However, watching too much TV can cause negative effects on health and well-being. Recently, public health efforts have largely aimed to influence and reduce TV usage and screen time.

Older adults and TV consumption

For various reasons, many older adults spend a considerable amount of their day watching television. In fact, adults aged 65 years or older spend threefold more time watching TV than younger and middle-aged adults [2]. Despite older adults watching more hours of TV than younger people, they seem to enjoy it less. Which begs the question, why do older people watch so much TV? This could be explained by older adults having fewer demands on their time than younger adults; for example, they no longer go to work every day. Watching TV allows them to spend time. This seems to be a significant factor in increasing screen time of older adults.

What is cognitive decline?

Cognition is the ability to make sense of the world around us. Cognition allows us to understand and respond appropriately to normal day-to-day events. Cognitive

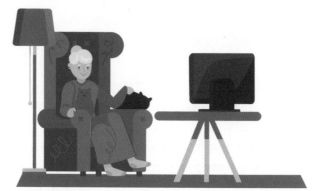

Older adults over 65 spend three times as many hours watching TV as younger adults

decline refers to the decreased ability to do this and is often considered a natural aspect of the ageing process. Cognitive decline can often manifest as forgetting things more frequently, losing a train of thought while in conversations, or having trouble navigating familiar areas or environments. Cognitive decline could also make it difficult to make decisions and understand instructions. However, cognitive decline can present differently in individuals and at varying rates, making it challenging to explain.

Cognitive decline is the first stage toward severe memory loss and, if it worsens, can lead to dementia and Alzheimer's. While the aetiology of dementia is still largely unknown, experts accept that individuals who remain engaged in mental activity are less affected by the cognitive decline of the ageing process than those who do not stay mentally active.

The passivity of TV Viewing

Compared to other sedentary forms of entertainment, such as reading, board games or paper-based brain games (sudoku, crosswords, etc.), TV is the most passive way of receiving stimuli. Unlike watching TV, these other forms of entertainment involve more interaction and can offer cognitive benefits such as problem-solving and enhanced visual-spatial skills. These are the skills we require to function in daily life. Rarely does watching TV require participation. The passivity of TV viewing and the increased hours spent in front of the television is considered to contribute to cognitive decline.

How much is too much TV?

Research carried out by Fancourt and team looked at television viewing habits and their association with cognition decline [3]. The study was carried out by researchers at the University College London and looked at data of over 3000 adults. The participants were asked to answer questions about their time spent watching television and were required to complete verbal memory and fluency tests. The analysis of this data revealed that the participants who watched television for 3.5 hours or more a day had around an 8-10% decline in language and word-related memory [3]. This is compared to a 4-5% decline amongst those participants who watched fewer hours of TV in the same period [3]. The results showed that watching TV for more than 3.5 hours daily is detrimental to memory function by almost doubling its decline.

The link between television and impairment of brain function is further supported by Hoang and team's study. The study looked at over 3000 adults over a 25-year period to assess television viewing and physical activity [4]. It identified high television viewing and low physical activity

as risk factors for cognitive impairment amongst middle-aged and older adults [4].

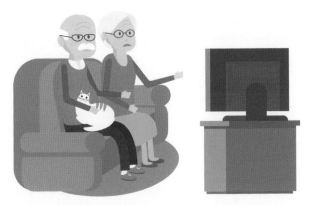

Watching high amounts of TV causes cognitive impairments and a greater decline in word-related memory

TV and cognitive stress

It is also important to note that it is not only how long we spend watching TV that could impact our cognitive function, but also the types of programmes we are watching. A lot of what is shown on TV, whether from news outlets or television programmes, is violent in nature and, for some, can be alarming. Violence and aggression are common themes in many popular TV shows, with the aim to interest and excite the viewer. However, Fancourt and team's study suggested that watching such psychologically distressing TV, with suspenseful, violent, and graphic scenes, may often cause "cognitive stress" [3]. "Cognitive stress" is essentially stress and tension in the mind. Stress increases the secretion of glucocorticoids, which are a class of steroid hormones that work in the fight-or-flight response. Glucocorticoids release glucose into the blood so that the body uses it for energy. When we are stressed, these steroid hormones are released, providing the glucose (sugar) needed to respond to the stressful stimuli. This is an evolutionary adaptation that humans have developed to escape predators or to engage in battle. In the past, exposure to stressful stimuli and the consequent release of stress hormones and glucose were necessary for the fight-or-flight response. The body reacts the same way when watching violent or graphic scenes on TV. Little does the body know that it is sat on a couch on a lazy Sunday afternoon watching the latest horror film. Therefore, the stress hormones which have been released needlessly and which have not been used cause the damage. The hippocampus is a vulnerable area of the brain embedded deep within the temporal lobe. It is responsible for memory [3]. Excessive and prolonged glucocorticoid exposure can lead to permanent damage in the hippocampus and lead to cognitive decline and memory loss

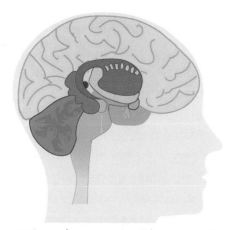

Excessive glucocorticoid exposure can damage the hippocampus, leading to cognitive decline and memory impairments

Inflammation is a natural response to infection or injury and is characterized by redness, swelling, fever and pain – it helps the body heal [5]. Inflammation can be measured in the body through

inflammatory markers. Inflammatory markers are certain proteins detectable in blood tests, which signify how much inflammation there is throughout the body. Therefore, when an individual is injured or fighting an infection, their inflammatory markers will temporarily rise but will reduce once they are better. This is what is known as acute inflammation. However, chronic inflammation, which is inflammation that is long-term and lasts for at least several months, is less understood. [5]. Mild, persistent chronic inflammation can cause irreversible organ dysfunction, as the body's response can lead to damage to healthy cells, organs, and tissues [5]. Chronic inflammation is linked to heart attacks, lung diseases, Type II diabetes and even cancer. Increased TV viewing is known to increase chronic inflammation. Research has shown that extended periods of television viewing can be linked to chronic inflammation.

A study by Grace and colleagues observed 8,933 adults for an average of 13.6 years [6]. They examined the participants' TV viewing habits and inflammatory-related mortality (death by cancer, cardiovascular disease etc.). The researchers found that every additional hour of TV time per day was associated with an increased risk of inflammatory-related death, even after factoring in smoking status, alcohol intake, diet and various other factors.

To conclude, there are three harmful effects that may be caused by prolonged periods of TV viewing. Firstly, of course, the more time spent sat watching TV, the more amount of time the body is sedentary. The health implications of excessive sedentary behaviour have been discussed in a previous chapter. Secondly, TV viewing, compared to other physically passive activities like using the computer or playing board games, causes cognitive decline due to the lack of any interactive or mental response required by the viewer.

Finally, too much TV may also lead to an increase in chronic inflammation, which can contribute towards conditions like cancer and cardiovascular disease, affecting the quality of life and life expectancy.

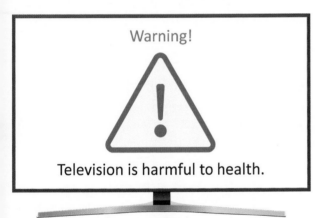

Warning!

Television is harmful to health.

Who has a social responsibility?

Despite the overwhelming research that shows the damage that can be caused by watching TV for prolonged periods of time, there are limited or rather no guidelines for how much TV should be watched a day.

An increase in public awareness is required, which could encourage people to participate in more active leisure pursuits and help decrease the negative effects of passive TV viewing. Thus, it could be suggested that socially conscious broadcasting companies, such as the BBC should provide statutory warnings to their viewers. Repeated and regular warnings may encourage viewers to decrease the time spent watching TV and seek other active leisure pursuits.

What can I do?

There is no denying that, in many instances, TV can be an effective tool of education and entertainment. However, individuals should be mindful of the adverse effects that too much TV can have. Simple measures like performing short spurts of exercises intermittently, for instance during advert breaks may break the physical passivity of watching TV and also provide some much-needed therapeutic exercises for the body. Another option is to watch TV in moderation and to interrupt it with physical activity. An hour of watching television could be followed by a walk.

Chapter 5 – What Is Arthritis?

Introduction

Arthritis is inflammation of the joints causing pain and disability. It can affect any joint, including the spine, hands, hips, knees, and ankles. The ends of bones which form joints are covered with smooth, white cartilage. This is called hyaline cartilage. This cartilage allows frictionless movement whilst providing strength to bear our weight. Unfortunately, hyaline cartilage is only produced once and cannot regenerate. Hence if hyaline cartilage is damaged, it cannot be replaced like for like. Following injury, it is replaced with fibrocartilage, which is inferior. Fibrocartilage is not as strong and does not have the frictionless weight-bearing properties of hyaline cartilage. It is, therefore, essential to keep the original hyaline cartilage healthy. Sadly, arthritis causes damage to this cartilage, causing significant pain, disability and affecting the quality of life.

Types of arthritis

There are many different variations of arthritis, each with its own causes and effects. The two main categories of the condition are labelled inflammatory arthritis and noninflammatory arthritis.

Inflammatory arthritis / rheumatoid arthritis / ankylosing spondylitis

An example of inflammatory arthritis is rheumatoid arthritis, a common condition affecting up to 1% of the population [1]. Women are twice more affected than men [1]. Rheumatoid arthritis is an autoimmune inflammatory disease where the body's immune system malfunctions, releasing enzymes that attack the lining and the surface of joints. Types of inflammatory arthritis, like rheumatoid arthritis, can affect many joints, including the wrists and fingers. The damage to the joints can lead to deformities. Other symptoms of inflammatory arthritis include fatigue, weight loss and fever [1]. The cardinal feature of autoimmune arthritis is early morning stiffness which resolves after an hour or two. The condition is treated through the use of anti-inflammatories or disease-modifying antirheumatic drugs (DMARDs). These medications block the enzymes that attack the joints, preventing further damage to the cartilage. Although such medications can reduce the effects of the condition, they often have many negative side effects, including stomach upset, liver damage and severe lung infections [1].

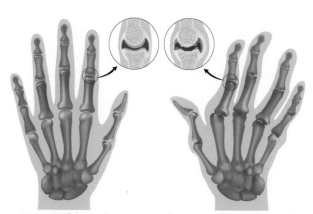

Normal hand   Hand with Rheumatoid Arthritis

Noninflammatory arthritis/osteoarthritis/ "wear and tear" arthritis

The most common example of noninflammatory arthritis is osteoarthritis. This is a progressive condition caused by wear and tear. In this form of arthritis, the smooth white cartilage at the ends of the bones is worn away. In advanced cases, the raw bones rub and grate against each other, reducing joint flexibility and producing pain in the affected area.

X-ray of the stages of Osteoarthritis of the knee

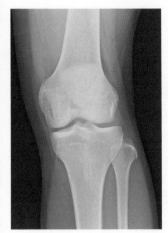 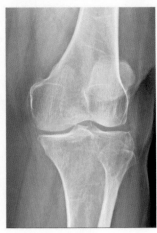 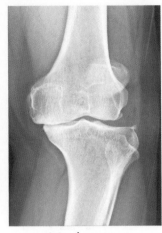 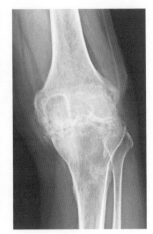

| Normal knee | Mild Osteoarthritis | Moderate Osteoarthritis | Severe Osteoarthritis |

Though it is termed wear and tear arthritis, it seems that osteoarthritis is not caused by "overuse" but rather "abuse". There is no evidence that participating in ordinary sporting activities or running regularly causes osteoarthritis. On the contrary, this may have a protective influence. There is, however, evidence that overloading joints as a result of obesity or significant joint injuries can result in osteoarthritis [2].

Patients who have this condition experience physical limitations. For instance, their ability to work or perform their household chores. Unfortunately, there is currently no effective medication to treat this type of arthritis. Medicines are only symptomatic, meaning they only control the pain. Nevertheless, exercising and reducing weight can help prevent and decrease the debilitating effects of osteoarthritis.

Illustration of knee Osteoarthritis and total knee replacement

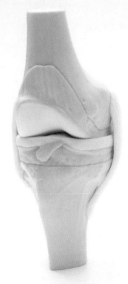 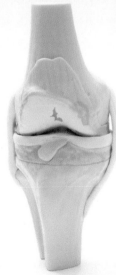 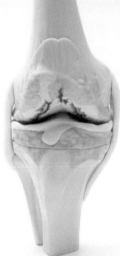 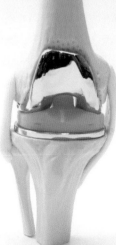

| Normal knee | Mild Osteoarthritis | Severe Osteoarthritis | Total knee replacement |

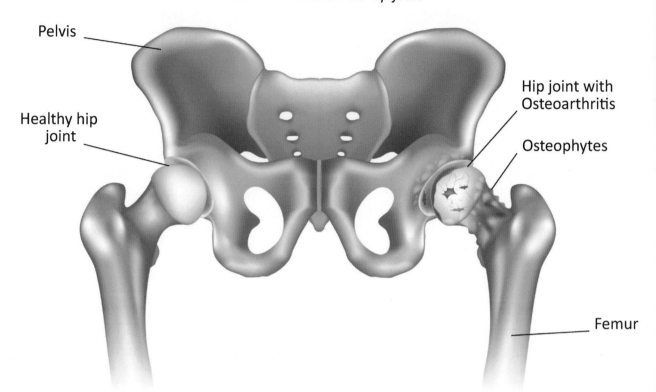

Normal and arthritic hip joint

Pelvis

Hip joint with Osteoarthritis

Healthy hip joint

Osteophytes

Femur

Normal hip joint   Hip joint with Osteoarthritis

Is surgery a good solution for hip arthritis?
Osteoarthritis of the knee and hip can be debilitating and affects a significant number of people. 25% of people will develop osteoarthritis of the hip in their lifetime [3]. The condition can cause severe pain and disability, and many patients may turn to surgery, in the form of a hip replacement, as treatment. A total hip replacement involves removing the diseased joint and replacing the joint with an artificial joint. Though these artificial joints are the best that man has made, it is a much inferior second compared to what nature provided originally. The estimated lifetime risk of undergoing a total hip replacement for end-stage osteoarthritis is 9% [3].

The popularity of total hip replacements is evident in the national statistics. Between 2017 and 2019, over 281,000 primary hip replacements were carried out in England, Wales and Northern Ireland [4]. Although necessary and effective for end-stage arthritis, a total hip replacement is a procedure that comes with a degree of risk. A study by Halawi and colleagues found that 11% of patients who underwent a total hip replacement reported unsatisfactory results. Of this 11%, 41% experienced persistent pain, and 35%

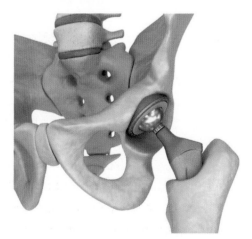

Total hip replacement

experienced physical limitations [5]. The risk of undergoing such surgery and the threat of associated unsatisfactory results highlights the importance of preventative measures and the need for other treatment options.

Is surgery a good solution for knee arthritis?

The story is the same, if not worse, regarding knee osteoarthritis. Between 2017 and 2019, over 310,000 knee replacement procedures were conducted in England, Wales, and Northern Ireland [4]. Although necessary and effective in most cases of end-stage arthritis, knee replacements, like hip replacements, come with some risks. One literature review indicated that around 20% of patients who undergo a total knee arthroplasty (replacement) report dissatisfaction following the procedure [6]. The researchers state that the most common reasons for dissatisfaction following the surgery include patients' overestimations of the potential benefits before the operation [6]. Over the last decade, this ratio of one dissatisfied patient for every five total knee replacements has been consistently observed, despite the positive developments in surgical technologies and treatments.

What to ask your doctor/surgeon before any intervention

These reports of disappointment, however, may not be the fault of the surgical procedure itself. They may arise due to a lack of communication or as a consequence of misinformation. The decision to undergo surgery should be a joint process between the surgeon and patient. The patient should be fully informed of the risks and benefits of both surgical and non-surgical treatments before agreeing to the procedure [7]. "Choosing Wisely" is a global initiative aimed at improving these discussions between patients and healthcare professionals. They state that the following four questions should be asked by patients to ensure they are fully informed about all aspects of their possible procedure [7]:

1. What are the benefits?
2. What are the risks?
3. What are the alternatives?
4. What if I do nothing?

Harm from arthroscopy

It should also be noted that some interventions, such as arthroscopy, do not always help and may make the condition worse. Arthroscopies are keyhole procedures during which an endoscope (a small camera) is inserted through a small incision to examine the state of the joint. This is conducted with the aim of examining the damage and washing out the joint. However, multiple randomised trials have shown that this small procedure is no more beneficial than placebo or sham procedures [8]. In addition, it may have adverse effects and can further damage the joint. Merely washing out and debriding the joint (removing the damaged pieces of cartilage) may sound logically wise, but in reality, it causes more harm. Consequently, performing an arthroscopy in a degenerate joint increases the risk of requiring a total knee replacement by three times [9].

Such statistics and facts highlight the need to avoid these interventions long before

Arthroscopy

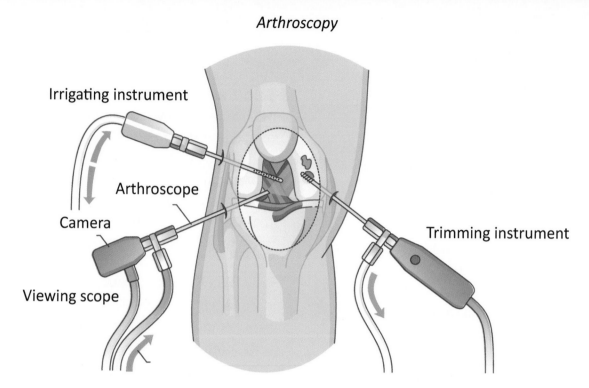

Irrigating instrument

Arthroscope

Camera

Viewing scope

Trimming instrument

they are necessary by reducing the occurrence of osteoarthritis through preventative measures.

What can be done?

Evidence-based lifestyle changes, such as weight loss and exercises, have been shown to decrease the occurrence of osteoarthritis and its associated symptoms. A systematic review by Charlesworth and team investigated the effects of different interventions on osteoarthritis. A systematic review is a research study that analyses the results of many other studies and combines them together. In Charlesworth's and colleagues review, lifestyle modifications (weight loss and exercise) were found to have benefits that lasted longer than 12 months, including reduced cartilage wear, and were highly recommended by the researchers due to their safety and effectiveness [10]. However, such treatments are not recommended enough and are often ignored in favour of

expensive and inefficient medications and injections [10]. For instance, cortisone (steroid) injections attempt to relieve pain and inflammation in a targeted area of the body. However, Charlesworth and team found that, though these injections have beneficial outcomes, they were also associated with increased cartilage wear, which may be counterproductive in the long run [10]. In addition, paracetamol and opioids are two of the most commonly prescribed medications for osteoarthritis, yet they are only as effective as placebo and can potentially cause harmful gastrointestinal (digestive system) complications when over-prescribed [10].

In summary

1. Aim to exercise regularly by walking to and from work, shops, school, church or social gatherings.
2. Aim for a healthy weight that will not overburden your joints.

Chapter 6 – Red Meat

Introduction

Red meat has become a common ingredient in human diets across the world. However, it may not be as good for humans as once thought. The term "red meat" encompasses beef, veal, pork, lamb, and mutton. The meat gets its red colour because of a chemical reaction. It contains high concentrations of myoglobin which, in the presence of oxygen, converts to oxymyoglobin. This is what gives the meat its reddish complexion [1]. The annual global production of red meat now stands at 184 million tonnes, 75 million tons more than poultry production [1]. Per capita consumption has also increased. The average daily intake is between 50 and 100 grams per person. An intake of more than 200 grams per day is considered high [2].

Processed red meat

There are two variations of red meat – processed and unprocessed. Processed red meat has undergone treatment like curing, smoking and salting to extend its shelf-life or improve its flavour. Preservatives are also added. Consequently, processed meat usually contains much more sodium and nitrates than unprocessed meat. Examples of processed red meat include sausages, ham, bacon and salami [1].

Is red meat the holy grail of protein?

The general assumption is that red meat is an excellent source of protein. Hence, it is promoted as a tool for building muscle and keeping fit. However, consider a bull, an elephant, a rhino or a gorilla. These animals are herbivores and consume only plant matter, yet they have vast amounts of muscle and immense strength. This indicates that meat is not the holy grail of protein we think it is.

Why can red meat be harmful?

Whilst red meat does contain vitamins, minerals and other nutrients, it may also contain additives and contaminants introduced during processing. Hormones and antibiotics used throughout meat production may also pollute the final product [1]. The resulting cocktail of chemicals can have profound adverse effects on health.

Red meat and cancer

Red meat is a potential carcinogen. Carcinogens are substances which encourage the formation of cancer in a process called carcinogenesis. A working

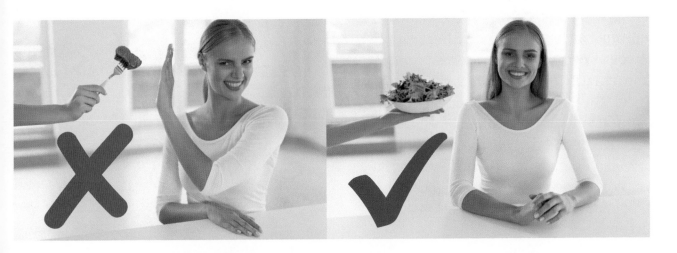

group of 22 scientists met in 2015 to evaluate the carcinogenicity of red meat and concluded that the evidence indicates that red meat consumption increases cancer risk [2]. Carcinogens, like the ones in red meat, can cause cancer by either disrupting metabolic processes or damaging the genetic material (genes and DNA). Damaging the genetic material can result in the development of cancer. One of the components of red meat is a form of iron called haem [1]. Haem plays a role in cancer development and is present in red meat at ten times the concentration in white meat [1]. Such high concentrations of haem in red meat result in an increased risk of cancer. Moreover, smoking the meat adds nitrates, which can increase the production of nitroso compounds within the bowels [1]. This greater concentration of nitroso compounds further increases the risk of developing cancer.

It should, however, be noted that carcinogens do not cause cancer in all circumstances or at all times. People are exposed to carcinogens every day, but it does not cause cancer. It is the repeated, intense exposure to the carcinogen that causes cancer. Smoking the first cigarette does not cause cancer, whilst smoking many cigarettes over a considerable period of time increases the risk. Even unprotected sunlight is a carcinogen. However, occasional unprotected sunlight exposure (UV light) will not cause skin cancer. On the other hand, repeated unprotected exposure to UV sunlight for extended periods may cause cancer. The same can be said for red meat – eating it occasionally over a lifetime will probably be fine, but repeated consumption causes adverse effects.

Based on a literature review, consumption of 50 grams of processed red meat per day increases the risk of breast cancer by 9% and both colorectoral and pancreatic cancer by 19% [1]. Even unprocessed red meat significantly increases the risk of cancers when consumed in higher amounts. For instance, consumption of 100 grams of unprocessed red meat per day can increase the risk of breast cancer by 11%, colon cancer by 17% and prostate cancer by 19% [1]. Development of lung, stomach, pancreas, liver, bladder and ovarian cancer is also linked to consumption of red meat.

The way we cook red meat can also increase its association with cancer. Cooking at high temperatures through pan-frying and barbecuing causes the production of harmful chemicals like heterocyclic amines (HAAs), polycyclic aromatic hydrocarbons (PAHs) and advanced glycation end products (AGEs). All these products are implicated with the increased risk of cancer [1].

Cancers associated with red meat

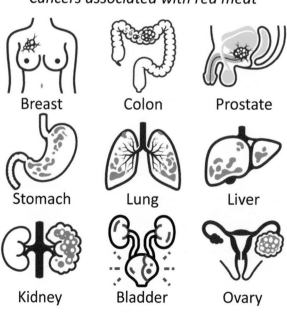

Breast	Colon	Prostate
Stomach	Lung	Liver
Kidney	Bladder	Ovary

Red meat and Type II diabetes (T2DM)

The consumption of red meat is associated with the development of Type II diabetes. Diabetes is defined as a metabolic disorder that causes a person's blood sugar level to rise to unhealthy levels. There are two types, Type I and Type II. Type I diabetes is an autoimmune disease where the body's immune system attacks and destroys cells that produce insulin, causing an insulin deficiency. This type is most commonly diagnosed in children and adolescents, though the condition can develop at any age. Type II diabetes is heavily associated with an unhealthy diet and lifestyle and can develop at any age, though it is most common in people over the age of 40. Symptoms of both variations include extreme thirst, fatigue, weight loss, and the occurrence of wounds that take a long time to heal. A meta-analysis by Feskens and team showed that the consumption of 50 grams of processed red meat increased the risk of developing Type II diabetes by 32% [3]. The study also showed that unprocessed red meat also increases the risk of developing Type II diabetes [3]. It is the high saturated fat content and the increased presence of iron (haem) found in red meat which contributes to the development of Type II diabetes. Whilst iron is essential for producing blood, too much is harmful. One study involving over 9000 participants showed that a high intake of dietary iron (haem) increased the risk of developing Type II diabetes [1].

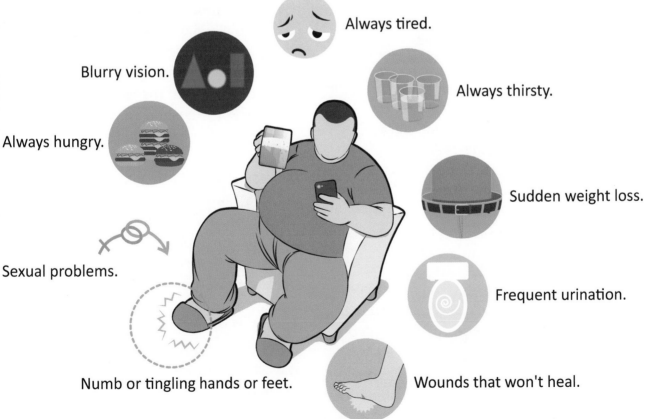

Symptoms of Diabetes

Always tired.

Blurry vision.

Always thirsty.

Always hungry.

Sudden weight loss.

Sexual problems.

Frequent urination.

Numb or tingling hands or feet.

Wounds that won't heal.

Red meat and cardiovascular diseases (CVD)

Cardiovascular diseases refer to conditions that narrow blood vessels. They include strokes caused by the decreased blood supply to the brain and coronary heart disease or heart failure caused by the decreased blood supply to the heart muscle.

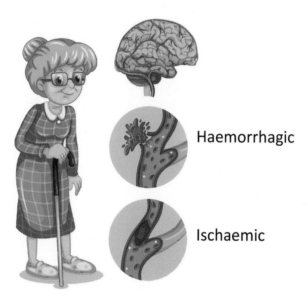

Common types of Stroke

1) Red meat and strokes

A stroke is a potentially life-threatening medical condition that occurs when the blood supply to part of the brain is blocked. When this occurs, the brain is starved of the oxygen and nutrients normally provided by the blood, resulting in the death of brain cells. This can cause permanent neurological impairment, disability or even death. There are two main types of stroke, ischemic and haemorrhagic. Ischemic strokes are caused by blood clots that cut off the blood supply to the brain, whereas haemorrhagic strokes result from a burst blood vessel supplying the brain. Red meat consumption has been linked to the occurrence of ischemic strokes in particular. For example, a community-based study in the U.S. by Haring and team assessed 11,601 adults over 22.7 years regarding stroke incidence. The results showed that consuming one serving per day of unprocessed and processed red meat increased the risk of stroke by 24% and 41%, respectively. [4].

2) Red meat and coronary heart disease (CHD)

Coronary arteries supply blood to the heart. Over time, fatty substances (cholesterol) stick to the walls within these arteries, interrupting the heart's blood supply. This results in chest pain, nausea and shortness of breath. Coronary heart disease is a leading cause of heart attacks and death in the UK and is associated with lifestyle factors, including smoking and drinking alcohol. Individuals are more at risk from coronary heart disease if they have high blood pressure, high cholesterol or diabetes. Increased risk of coronary heart disease has also been related to red meat consumption. The Nurses Health Study by Bernstein and co-workers investigated this and included 84,136 women aged between 30 and 55 years. The results showed that consumption of red meat caused a significantly increased risk of coronary heart disease compared to consumption of poultry, fish and nuts [5]. A separate analysis of six studies further investigated the effects of processed meat (both white and red) on coronary heart disease. The results showed that every 50 grams serving/day of processed meat was associated with a 42% higher risk of the condition [1].

3) Red meat and heart failure

Heart failure occurs when the heart muscle is unable to pump blood as well as it should. This can be caused by narrowed arteries within the heart (atherosclerosis) or by high blood pressure. These conditions can leave the heart too weak or stiff to pump blood efficiently, resulting in breathlessness, tiredness and dizziness. A population-based prospective study from Sweden, which included 34,057 participants, showed that consumption of 50 g per day of processed red meat increased the risk of heart failure in women by 11% [6].

All-cause mortality

All-cause mortality refers to death from any cause. A meta-analysis including more than 1.3 million people from nine prospective studies (five from the U.S., three from Europe and one from China) showed that red meat consumption caused increased all-cause mortality [7]. This study also assessed how this risk was increased depending on the amount of red meat consumed. Consuming 60 grams of red meat per day increased the risk of death by 22%, when compared to a smaller daily intake of 10 grams [7].

What can be done?

Adopting a vegetarian diet may help reduce the risk of the conditions associated with red meat consumption. Even substituting the red meat with poultry or fish is advantageous. It may be difficult to suddenly cut out the red meat from a diet entirely. Therefore, it is recommended that individuals attempt to gradually reduce their red meat intake over time until they consume none at all. By removing red meat from diets completely, individuals may be able to live longer and happier lives.

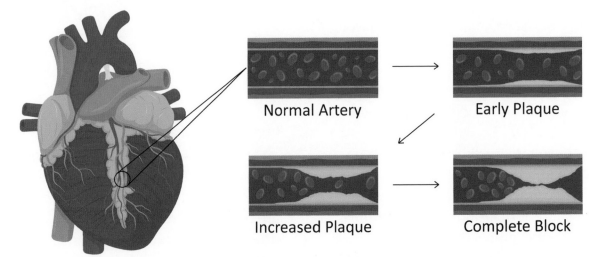

Stages of narrowing of the Coronary Artery supplying the Heart

Chapter 7 – Dairy

Introduction

Dairy has garnered a reputation for being high in calcium. Calcium is an important mineral that helps keep our bones strong while also regulating muscle contractions, such as the heartbeat. As a result, dairy and milk products have become staples in human diets across the world and now account for around 14% of the caloric intake in developed countries [1]. Unsurprisingly, since 1988 global milk production has increased by 60%, from 530 million tons to around 843 million tons, to meet a growing demand [2]. However, questions are now being raised regarding how beneficial dairy calcium is to our overall health.

The calcium myth

Although calcium is necessary for bone health, the body can only absorb a limited amount. In fact, the body can take in just 32% of the calcium within dairy products [3]. So, if a person drinks a cup of milk that contains 300 milligrams of calcium per cup, only around 96 milligrams will be absorbed and utilised by the body. In comparison, the body can consume a lot more of the calcium found in leafy greens. For instance, up to 60% of the calcium found in broccoli is absorbable [3]. This means that if a person consumes one cup of broccoli, which contains around 70 milligrams of calcium, 43 milligrams will be absorbed and used by the body [3]. Bok choy, which is an Asian cabbage that can be found in some UK supermarkets, can provide even more useable calcium. A cup of bok choy has a calcium content of around 160 milligrams, of which 85 milligrams (54%) can be absorbed [3]. Therefore, eating one cup of bok choy provides almost as much absorbable calcium as drinking one cup of milk whilst also providing many other essential vitamins and minerals.

The lack of calcium absorbability in milk may help to explain the findings of one literature review conducted by Bian and team in 2018. They looked at the results of 18 previous studies which had investigated the effects of dairy consumption on bone fracture risk [4]. The review found that consuming 200 grams of milk a day did not reduce hip fracture risk, suggesting that consuming a lot of milk, which many people may do to enhance bone health, may do nothing to improve bone integrity [4].

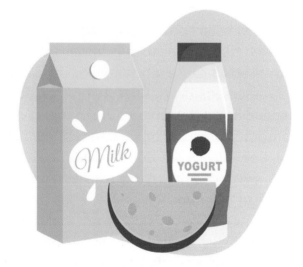

The body can only absorb around a third of the calcium found in dairy products

Lactose Intolerance

To process dairy products, humans need to have a specific enzyme called lactase. This enzyme is vital in the digestion of dairy as it breaks down the lactose within it. However, most people (around 65% globally) do not have this enzyme, which is

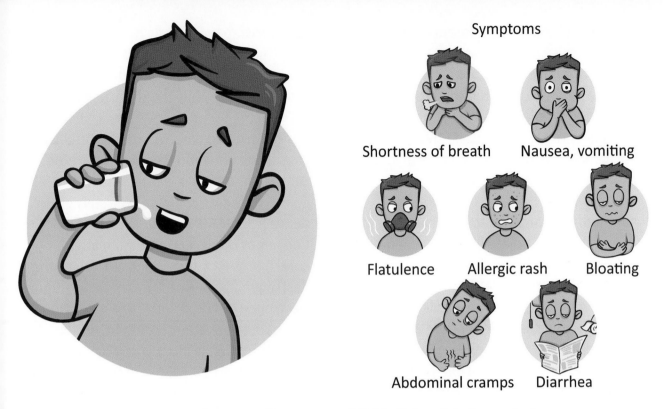

Symptoms

Shortness of breath

Nausea, vomiting

Flatulence

Allergic rash

Bloating

Abdominal cramps

Diarrhea

Lactose intolerance affects around 65% of the global population

lost after childhood. These individuals are called "lactose intolerant" and may experience flatulence and diarrhoea after eating dairy. Lactose intolerance is a common digestive problem, and the lack or shortage of the lactase enzyme makes the body unable to digest dairy. Therefore, dairy consumption is not entirely natural for most of the world, which is inconsistent with the current consumption levels. Man is the only animal to drink milk into adulthood. Hence one has to wonder if drinking milk is a natural process. So, what kind of effects does consuming dairy have on us?

Cardiovascular disease

Cardiovascular disease is a major cause of morbidity globally. Diet is largely associated as a crucial aspect of its pathology and prevention. Dairy products, such as cheese, milk, butter, yoghurt and ice cream, are high in saturated fat and cholesterol. Diets high in saturated fat can increase the risk of heart disease and other serious health issues.

Cancer

Consumption of dairy products has been heavily linked to an increased risk of various cancers. In a 2013 study, 21,660 participants were observed over a period of 28 years. Information regarding their dairy consumption was collected at baseline, and the number of prostate cancer cases and deaths were reported at follow-up [5]. The researchers found that men who consumed 2.5 or more servings of dairy products a day had an increased risk of prostate cancer than those who consumed half a serving or less [5]. Similar research findings have been found in countries all over the world, such as Canada and Japan, showing that the correlation is unlikely to be affected by demographics [5].

The same study then carried out a second piece of analysis. They took the patients who had developed prostate cancer during the study period and noted the type of milk (skimmed or whole milk) they consumed. The researchers then assessed these participants' prostate cancer survival rates in order to observe any associations between survival and the type of milk consumed. The analysis found that the consumption of whole milk was related to a higher risk of fatal prostate cancer, with lower survival rates [5]. On the contrary, skimmed milk consumption was linked to nonaggressive disease (low-grade and early-stage cases) and improved survival rates [5]. This indicates that the type of milk consumed can make a considerable difference in cancer-mortality risks.

Due to the association identified between dairy intake and a higher risk of both developing and dying from prostate cancer, questions have been raised about whether dairy should be considered a part of a balanced diet and whether regular consumption of milk should be recommended, especially for older men?

These links between dairy consumption and some cancers are probably, at least partially, related to increases in the insulin-like growth factor (IGF-1) found in cow's milk. IGF-1 has been heavily associated with prostate cancer, as men with high levels have been found to be over four times more likely to develop the disease than those with low IGF-1 levels [6]. Due to IGF-1 being found in cow's milk, research has questioned whether there could be a causal link between dairy consumption and cancer growth. This is also true regarding colon cancer, as colon-cancer cells grow faster from IGF-1 exposure [7]. Consumption of milk and dairy also contributes to a significant portion of the oestrogen intake in a human diet. Oestrogen is linked with cancers of the reproductive system, including breast and ovarian cancer. A large study by Fraser and team included 52,795 women who were followed for almost eight years. Dairy consumption habits and the number of cancer cases were assessed throughout this period to see if there was any causal relationship. The study found that higher intakes of dairy milk were associated with a 50% increase in breast cancer risk [8]. Furthermore, the ten-year Iowa Women's Health Study of more than 29,000 premenopausal women found that women who consumed one glass or more of milk each day had a 73% greater chance of developing ovarian cancer than women who drank less than one glass a day [9].

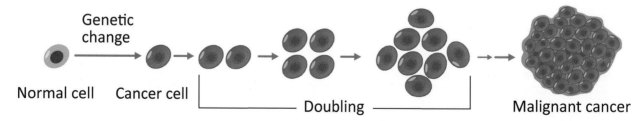

Cow's milk contains insulin-like growth factor (IGF-1) which is heavily associated with cancer tumour growth

Diabetes is a chronic disease that can cause an individual's blood sugar level to become too high. Over half the number of those living with diabetes in the UK today are aged over 65 years old, which shows that it is a considerable problem for those in their later years of life.

While Type II diabetes is more common, research has found that dairy consumption can influence the development of both variations. Type I diabetes is associated with the consumption of dairy products during infancy. The American Academy of Paediatrics produced a policy statement regarding this in 2012. It stated that, based on the data available, infants who are breastfed in the first three months of their lives are 30% less likely to be diagnosed with Type I diabetes [10]. Breastfeeding is thought to reduce this risk, as it enables infants to avoid exposure to the adverse effects of cow's milk protein [10]. The paper also reports that being breastfed for the first three months of life reduces the risk of Type II diabetes by 40% [10]. In addition, a similarly high reduction is identified regarding breastfeeding and obesity. Infants who are breastfed at any occurrence during their infancy have a 15-30% reduction in obesity in their adolescent and older adult years [10].

What can you do?

So, despite dairy being a key ingredient for many of the meals and recipes we eat daily, research tells us that dairy consumption may have adverse effects on health. It can promote the development of many conditions, including cardiovascular disease and cancers. If individuals wish to avoid such diseases, they should reconsider the amount of dairy they want to consume, especially given that dairy products may not be as beneficial for bone health as assumed.

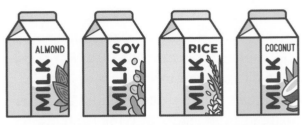

There are many alternatives available to dairy milk, including almond milk, soy milk, rice milk and coconut milk

As this information becomes more widespread, and in an attempt to live a more environmentally friendly life, many individuals are now swapping their dairy products for low/non-fat or plant-based alternatives. More dairy alternative products are available on the market than ever before, meaning that you can enjoy the same foods and tastes without adverse health risks. The most popular of these substitutes include soy cheeses, plant-based yoghurt and coconut, almond, soy and rice milk.

Chapter 8 – Food from Plants

Introduction

Vegetarianism is becoming more common as people realise the health and environmental benefits of reducing meat consumption. However, vegetarianism is not a modern concept. The idea that plant-based diets are better than meat-based diets is even highlighted in books as old as the Bible. In the story of Daniel and his three friends, four young captives in Babylon were chosen by the king to be his advisors. The young men accepted this way of life in every sense – except for the diet of the king. They refused to eat the royal food and wine and instead chose a diet of vegetables and water. This surprised the king's officers, and Daniel suggested a ten-day trial as a compromise. Daniel and his friends ate their plant-based diet for the duration of the trial, while the other advisors enjoyed the royal food. The scripture states, "At the end of the ten days, Daniel and his friends looked healthier and more nourished than the other young men who ate the royal food" (Daniel 1:15). This may be the first controlled experiment recorded in human history.

This story, although over 2500 years old, highlights the benefits of a plant-based diet. Additionally, early medicine revolved around the prescription of vegetables and fruits as medicine to prevent diseases.

The Adventist philosophy

The Seventh-Day Adventist Church of Loma Linda has linked theology and food to encourage a vegetarian lifestyle amongst believers. Followers of the Seventh Day Adventist church believe their bodies are holy temples which should only be fed the healthiest foods. As a result, they began mass-producing their own plant-based foods, including meat alternatives, breakfast cereals and soy milk. Dr John Harvey Kellogg (February 26, 1852 – December 14, 1943), an American doctor, was a Seventh-Day Adventist. He prescribed vegetarian food to his patients and introduced Kellogg's plant-based cereals as breakfast for the whole world.

The Adventist Health Studies are long-term studies investigating the correlations between lifestyle, diet and disease among members of the Adventist church. One of these, a 2013 study by Orlich and colleagues, involved 73,308 members of the Adventist church. The investigation compared the mortality rates of vegetarian church members vs. non-vegetarian church members regarding various health conditions. The study found

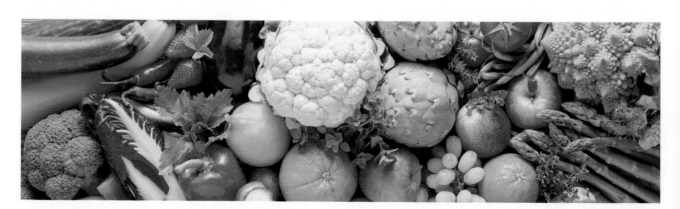

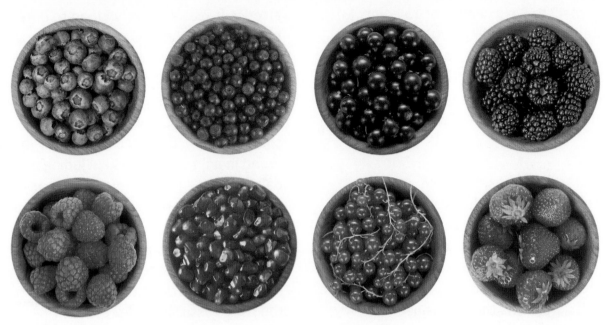

Berries have a low Glycemic Index (less sugar) and are a healthy choice of fruits

that individuals who follow vegetarian diets had a 13% lower risk of dying from cardiovascular diseases, an 8% reduction in risk of dying from cancer and a 29% reduced risk of dying due to endocrine diseases (e.g. diabetes). The paper also concluded that vegetarian diets lower all-cause mortality, or death by any means, by around 12% [1].

The benefits of plant-based diets

Reducing the symptoms of osteoarthritis
A study conducted by Clinton and colleagues investigated the effectiveness of a plant-based diet in reducing the symptoms of osteoarthritis [2]. Patients with osteoarthritis were randomised into two groups. One group was provided with information regarding plant-based diets available from https://www.pcrm.org/, and the other group followed their regular normal diet. The study ran concurrently for a period of six weeks. Participants in the plant-based diet group increased their energy and physical functionality by 10%

[2]. Additionally, following the second week of the experiment, the vegan participants experienced less pain in the joints that were arthritic [2].

Various fact sheets and recipes are freely available from the PCRM (Physicians Committee for Responsible Medicine) website at: https://pcrm.widencollective.com/portals/gr0kpkol/factsheets

Reducing the symptoms of rheumatoid arthritis
Diets rich in fibre, fruit and vegetables have anti-inflammatory properties and have been found to help reduce pain and inflammation in rheumatoid arthritis patients. A study by McDougall and colleagues investigated the effects of a vegan diet on patients with rheumatoid arthritis [3]. The results of the study showed that there were significant reductions in many symptoms. For instance, the degree of pain felt by the participants went down from an average

score of 49 to 34, a change of 15 points [3]. Limitations in the ability to function also decreased from 47 to 29, a decrease of 18 points [3]. Furthermore, the joint swelling score was reduced from a mean of 24 points to 17 points: a reduction of 7 points [3].

Cholesterol and heart disease

Cholesterol is one of the fats found in the blood. It is essential and required to build healthy cells. However, high levels of bad cholesterol can collect on the walls of arteries in a process known as atherosclerosis. As the excess bad cholesterol accumulates on the inside of arteries (tubes that carry blood to different body organs), the flow of blood through these arteries is restricted. This can increase the threat of strokes and heart disease. Food from plants is typically low in saturated fat and does not contain cholesterol [4]. Dietary cholesterol is only found in animal products, including meat, dairy and eggs [5]. Therefore, a meat-free diet can significantly reduce cholesterol concentrations, decreasing the risk of heart disease by about 10% [5]. Plant-based diets can also reverse atherosclerosis, thereby making the arteries clearer and reducing the risk of associated diseases [4].

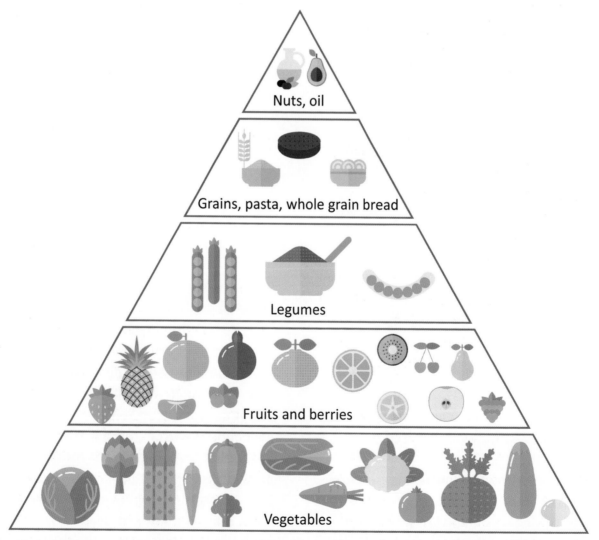

Plant Based Food Pyramid. A good diet should include a mix with more from the lower end of the pyramid.

Platelet aggregation

Platelet aggregation refers to the accumulation of platelets in the blood. Platelets are cells in the blood which help form clots to prevent bleeding. However, when these cells clump up within the arteries, as is the case in platelet aggregation, it can cause clots. These clots can block arteries and cause strokes and heart attacks [5]. Plant-based diets have been shown to reduce platelet aggregation and therefore decrease the threat of strokes and heart attacks [5]. Therefore, people who follow plant-based diets are 32% less likely to experience a coronary heart disease event and 29% less likely to experience a cerebral vascular disease event (stroke) [5]. The most effective foods for lowering risk include grains, vegetables, nuts and some fruits [5].

Furthermore, plant-based diets have also been shown to decrease insulin resistance, which has also been shown to help with metabolic syndrome. Metabolic syndrome is a combination of obesity, high blood pressure and Type II Diabetes [5]. Insulin resistance refers to the body's incapability to react to the same amount of insulin.

With insulin resistance, more and more insulin is needed to perform the same task. This is what happens in Type II Diabetes.

Blood pressure

Studies have shown that a plant-based diet can significantly reduce blood pressure [5]. Blood pressure is the force that your heart uses to pump blood around the body. A blood pressure measurement involves two readings – for example, a healthy blood pressure reading would be 120/80. The higher of the two values is called the systolic and is the pressure in the artery when the heart is contracting. The lower of the two values is called the diastolic and is the pressure in the artery when the heart is not contracting. High blood pressure, where these numbers would be larger than the healthy reading, is heavily linked with a greater risk of stroke, coronary heart disease and diabetes [5]. Thankfully, plant-based diets have been shown to reduce death by coronary heart disease by 7% and death by stroke by 14% [5]. Conversely, high protein intake from meat has been shown to increase blood pressure, further indicating the benefits of

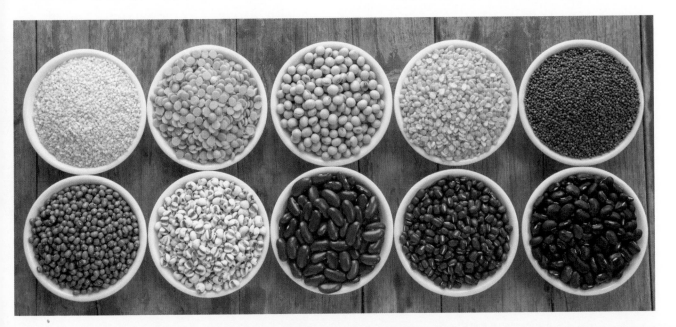

following a vegan/vegetarian diet [5]. Additionally, vegetarian diets are high in potassium, which has been revealed to decrease blood pressure further [5].

Type II diabetes

Type II diabetes is a metabolic disorder that makes a person's blood sugar levels rise too high, caused by a lack of effective insulin being produced. Insulin is a hormone made in the pancreas, which enables the glucose in the blood to enter the cell to be used as fuel. Insulin is like the oil tanker that delivers fuel to the petrol garages, moving the glucose from the blood into the cell. The insulin deficiency caused by the underperforming pancreas leaves too much glucose in the blood, resulting in high blood sugar levels. Whilst the worldwide prevalence of the condition is increasing overall, Type II diabetes prevalence is significantly lower in vegans and vegetarians than in meat-eaters [5].

Additionally, plant-based diets can prevent Type II diabetes and may be used as a treatment, as they have been shown to improve blood sugar control in patients with the condition [5]. Type II diabetes increases the risk of heart attacks and stroke. Hence resorting to a vegetarian/vegan diet and reducing the risk of Type II diabetes reduces the risk of heart attacks and stroke [5].

Overweight and obesity

Obesity is a massive health concern throughout the world. In the UK, according to published figures in 2020, 67% of men and 59% of women were overweight or obese [6]. Fortunately, plant-based diets can help with weight reduction. For instance, studies have shown that

participants can lose an average of two kilograms of body weight over 18 weeks following a vegan or vegetarian diet [5]. Additionally, vegetarians seem to have increased resting metabolism allowing them to lower their weight more quickly than non-vegetarians [5]. Thus, in addition to reducing weight, it maintains the BMI (Body Mass Index) at a healthy level. The BMI is calculated by dividing the weight in kilograms by the square of the height in meters. A person who weighs 70 kilograms (11 stone) and is 175 centimetres tall (five feet and eight inches) has a BMI of 22.85. This is calculated as follows,

$$BMI = \text{weight in kilograms}/(\text{Height in meters})^2 = 70/(1.75 \times 1.75) = 22.85.$$

It is ideal to maintain a BMI of 18.5 to 25. A BMI between 25 and 30 is considered overweight and above 30 is obese. A BMI above 40 is considered extremely obese.

What can be done?

Simply cutting down on the amount of meat consumed and increasing plant-based foods can contribute to better health. Attempt a gradual reduction of meat consumption and eventually, you may be able to cut it out completely. Salads and boiled vegetables should be the major portion of any meal.

Where will I get my protein?

One of the concerns is that, without meat, it is difficult to get the proper amounts of protein. However, plant-based foods contain more protein than is widely thought. In 2010, the U.S. Dietary Guidelines Advisory Committee reported that individuals consuming plant-based protein can still meet their protein requirements, despite consuming less meat [7]. Amazingly, three to four tablespoonfuls of nuts contain the same amount of protein as 100 grams of meat or 140 grams of fish [7].

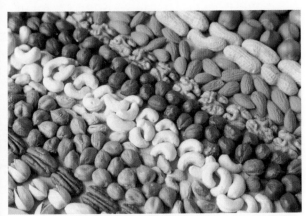

Nuts are rich in minerals, healthy fat and proteins

To investigate this, a study by Li and colleagues compared changes in the muscle size in people who ate plant-based protein with people who consumed animal protein. They found that both groups of people who ate plant-based or animal protein increased skeletal muscle mass [8]. This shows that protein from plants is just as effective as protein from meats in maintaining the size of our muscles [8].

Chapter 9 – Natural Alternatives to Medicine

Introduction

A natural alternative to medicine is usually food, which can either replace or complement the use of traditional medicines, such as ibuprofen and paracetamol. There are many different forms of natural alternatives and many different ways to consume them. For example, throughout history, spices and herbs have been used for culinary and medicinal purposes. Such foods are well known for their ability to enhance the flavour and smell of food whilst also providing colour and increasing shelf-life. However, herbs and spices have also been shown to protect us from acute and chronic diseases [1]. There is now an abundance of evidence that shows how many herbs and spices have anti-inflammatory, antioxidant, anticarcinogenic and cholesterol-lowering properties. Many of these can be beneficial for health [1]. Other food groups which can offer such protection include seeds, nuts and legumes (beans, peas etc.).

Examples of foods that can act as natural alternatives to medicine

The most beneficial foods which serve as natural alternatives to medicine include:

1. Sesame
2. Ginger
3. Turmeric
4. Garlic
5. Fibre
6. Nuts
7. Beans

1) Sesame

a) **Osteoarthritis:** Existing evidence suggests that sesame and its derivative sesame oil have anti-inflammatory properties that may aid in treating and managing osteoarthritis. A study involving 104 patients with knee osteoarthritis were asked to apply either 1.5 ml of sesame oil or diclofenac gel (an anti-inflammatory drug) three times a day for four weeks. The study concluded that the sesame oil reduced osteoarthritic knee pain more than the gel while also beneficial in other areas, including joint function [2].

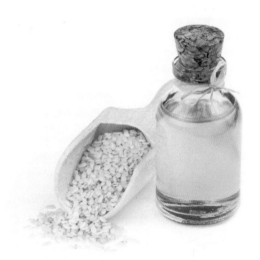

b) **Other inflammatory diseases:** A literature review published in 2019 investigated the effects of sesame on numerous other inflammatory diseases. The study concluded that sesame can stop the activity of inflammatory cytokines and mediators. Inflammatory cytokines are chemicals in the body that cause cell inflammation. Inflammation can be likened to a fire. A slow-burning fire is necessary to keep us warm, but a large fire can destroy and kill.

Similarly, some inflammation is required, but excessive inflammation in the body can be harmful. Sesame decreases inflammation and reduces the impact of inflammatory diseases like inflammatory bowel disease, lung disease, liver disease, and arthritis [2].

2) **Ginger**
   a) **Osteoarthritis:** Osteoarthritis, though a degenerative condition, is accompanied by inflammation. Decreasing inflammation in the joint is one of the modes of treatment. Tumour necrosis factor-α (TNF-α) and interleukin-1β (I.L.- 1β) are inflammatory markers in the body, and levels of these markers in the blood rise during inflammation. In a randomised control clinical trial, participants with osteoarthritis of the knee were either provided with capsules containing 500 milligrams of ginger powder or starch (a placebo) for three months [1]. Levels of these inflammatory markers were tested at the start and at the end of the study after three months. At the beginning of the study, there was no difference in the level of these inflammatory markers in both groups. At the end of the study, after three months, the group that consumed ginger saw a significant fall in the level of inflammatory markers [1]. This shows that oral consumption of ginger reduces the inflammation associated with osteoarthritis [1].

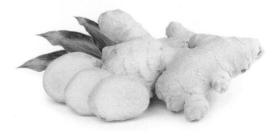

   b) **Cardiovascular health:** Lipids (fat in the blood) are crucial for a healthy heart. The fats that are usually measured in the blood are triglycerides, high-density lipoprotein cholesterol (HDL) and low-density lipoprotein cholesterol (LDL). High-density lipoprotein cholesterol is good fat, while triglycerides and low-density lipoprotein cholesterol are bad fats. In a randomised control trial, 85 patients were divided into two groups. The test group was provided with three grams of ginger as ginger capsules, and the control group was provided with a placebo. The trial continued for a period of 45 days [1]. Lipid levels at the start of the study were similar in both groups. When the lipid levels were retested at the end of the study in 45 days, the group that had three grams of ginger daily had decreased levels of the bad fats (triglycerides and low-density lipoprotein cholesterol) and higher levels of the good fat (high-density lipoprotein cholesterol) [1].

   c) **Weight-management:** The consumption of ginger can also help with weight management. Obesity is a huge concern in today's society. Consumption of ginger may help in weight reduction through two different modes of action. It increases satiety and increases heat generation. Increasing satiety increases the feeling of fullness and decreases the hunger and the need to eat. Increased heat generation from the spiciness of ginger causes body temperature to rise and increases metabolism. In one cross-over trial, ten overweight or obese men were initially given two grams of dried ginger with hot water with their morning breakfast [1]. In the second part of the trial, the same participants were provided with a normal breakfast without a drink of ginger. On the days when the participants consumed a hot drink with ginger, they showed a lack of appetite (increased satiety) and increased heat generation [1]. In another randomised control trial, 80 obese women were divided into two groups. The test group was given two grams of dried ginger, and the control group was given corn starch. Over the course of three months, the group provided with ginger decreased their BMI by 0.5 and reduced their insulin levels and HOMA IR index [1]. BMI is a measure of body composition where the body weight is divided by the square of the height in meters. One of the issues in diabetes and obesity is insulin resistance. Insulin resistance is where increased levels of insulin are required to perform the same task. HOMA IR is a method used to determine insulin resistance.

3) **Turmeric**
   a) **Osteoarthritis:** The active compound within turmeric is curcumin. Curcumin has anti-inflammatory properties, which can inhibit the effects of pro-inflammatory markers, helping maintain healthy joint function [1]. In a randomised control trial, 107 patients were randomly divided into two groups. The test group was provided with two grams of turmeric per day, and the control group was provided with 800 milligrams of ibuprofen [1]. The participants were assessed with regard to pain relief. Their time taken while level-walking 100 metres and climbing up and down a flight of stairs was also observed. At follow-up, there was no difference between the groups showing that two grams of turmeric was as effective as 800 milligrams of Ibuprofen in providing pain relief. There was also no difference in the adverse effects between the two groups [1].

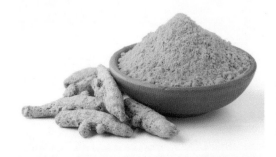

   b) **Healthy brain and maintaining cognition:** Curcumin can also help maintain healthy brain function in later life. A study in Singapore involving over 1000 participants aged between 60 and 93 showed that regular turmeric intake helped preserve cognitive function, even when only consumed occasionally [1]. More evidence for this was provided in another study, which found that participants who consumed 1500 milligrams of curcumin every day for 12 months had fewer declines in cognitive function than participants who received a placebo [1].

c) **Cardiovascular health and lipids:** Curcumin may also help with regard to cardiovascular health. One study showed that 500 milligrams of Curcumin per day for only seven days decreased patients' levels of bad cholesterol by as much as 12% while increasing good cholesterol levels by 29% [1].

4) **Garlic**
   a) **Osteoarthritis:** Garlic also has anti-inflammatory properties. In a randomised control trial, 76 overweight or obese women were randomised to receive either 1000 milligrams of odourless garlic tablets per day (equivalent to 2500 milligrams of raw garlic) or a placebo for 12 weeks. Pain, function and stiffness improved in the garlic group, but only the reduction in stiffness was statistically significant [1].

   b) **Cardiovascular health:** Garlic can also promote cardiovascular health [1]. Evidence from human trials

shows that garlic may help reduce fat formation and plaque within the blood vessels, thereby slowing or halting the development of atherosclerosis. Atherosclerosis is a process where the arteries become hardened and narrowed, leading to an increased risk of heart attacks and strokes [1]. In a randomised control trial, 92 overweight or obese participants were randomised to receive either 400 milligrams of garlic extract or a placebo for three months. The stiffness of the arteries (measured by the arterial stiffness index), the inflammation (measured by high sensitive C reactive protein) and the bad cholesterol (measured by LDL Cholesterol) were significantly lowered in the garlic group as compared to the placebo control group [1].

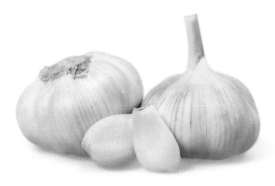

c) **Type II Diabetes:** Garlic consumption may also benefit patients with Type II diabetes. One investigation found that garlic supplementation significantly reduced glucose levels in the blood of Type II Diabetes patients over 24 weeks, therefore aiding in the management of the disease [1].

5) Dietary fibre

Dietary fibre refers to non-digestible plant-based carbohydrates which cannot be broken down by the body's digestive enzymes [3]. They are passed down into the large intestine, where it is broken down by the gut bacteria (microbiome – see Chapter 7). According to the American Diabetic Association, evidence shows that dietary fibre from whole foods or supplements may reduce the risk of diabetes as it improves the body's ability to process and use sugar after food consumption [3]. The association also says that fibre can decrease the risk of cardiovascular disease as it helps reduce cholesterol. For instance, increasing soluble fibre intake by five to ten grams daily is associated with a 5% reduction in bad cholesterol [3].

Additionally, diets high in fibre are associated with decreases in waist circumference, weight, and visceral adipose tissue [3]. Visceral adipose tissue is fat tissue located deep within the abdomen around the organs. It increases the risk of diabetes, cardiovascular disease, and some cancers. High dietary intakes of fruit and vegetables which contain fibre are associated with a reduced risk of cancer. Studies have shown a 10% reduction in the risk of colorectal cancer and a 7% reduction in the risk of breast cancer for every ten grams of fibre daily [3].

A prospective, multicentre cohort of 4,796 men and women aged between 45–79 years and at risk of developing osteoarthritis were followed up for 8 years. Increased fibre intake was associated with decreased knee pain and improved function. For adults, the current recommendation for fibre intake is 25–35 grams per day [3].

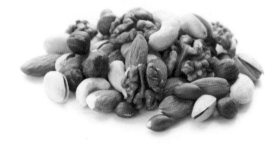

6) Nuts

Evidence suggests that a higher intake of nuts can lower the risk of death due to their antioxidant and anti-inflammatory properties [4]. Studies have shown that high consumption of nuts can reduce the risk of contracting diabetes by 26% and may reduce the risk of dying from the condition by as much as 32% [4]. Additionally, several studies indicated that participants who consumed the highest amount of tree nuts and peanuts were 40% less likely to die from any form of cancer than those who consumed the lowest number of nuts [4]. Furthermore, consuming at least one serving of walnuts a week can reduce the threat of cardiovascular disease by 17%, stroke by 17% and coronary heart disease by 21% [4]. Consumption of walnuts is also associated with better cognitive functioning and working memory in elderly populations [4]. Pistachios are also beneficial for health as they contain fibre, protein, unsaturated fatty acids, and many vitamins. All of these contribute to good health. Pistachios also contain high levels of melatonin [5]. Melatonin is a chemical that helps regulate the body's biological sleep and wake cycle, promoting good sleep [5]. Taking ten kernels of pistachios an hour-and-a-half before bed can help encourage a good night's sleep.

7) Beans

Beans are rich in fibre and antioxidants while low in sugar [6]. They can therefore have many health benefits. For instance, in both patients with and without diabetes, beans have been shown to reduce glucose levels, aiding in the management and prevention of the condition [6]. Additionally, although there is only a little evidence, beans may reduce the threat of pancreatic cancer [6]. In another study of nearly 10,000 men and women, bean intake was associated with reduced cardiovascular and coronary heart disease risk. A further study showed that the consumption of 120 grams of beans a day lowers bad cholesterol levels without affecting good cholesterol levels [6]. This is likely due to the soluble fibre content of beans, which is thought to decrease bad cholesterol [6]. Bean consumption also reduced inflammation, further decreasing the risk of cardiovascular disease and other health conditions associated with inflammation [6].

What can be done?

Add these ingredients while cooking to receive the benefits and potentially reduce reliance on medicines. Garlic, turmeric and ginger can be added to curries or pasta dishes. A turmeric latte can be made by adding turmeric and sugar to warm soya or almond milk. The recipe for this is provided at the end of this chapter. Consuming this latte a couple of hours before bedtime, along with a small handful of pistachio nuts, can provide both pain relief and restful sleep. It is also recommended that individuals attempt to replace crisps and other snacks with nuts. Furthermore, beans can be added to breakfast or in Mexican dishes. Having a healthy balanced diet with all these foods can keep many diseases and health problems at bay.

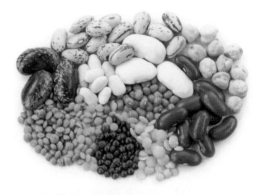

How to make a Turmeric Latte

Take an ordinary teacup and fill it with 50 millilitres of milk. The cup should be only 1/4th full. Use plant-based milk (soya, almond or oats) if possible.

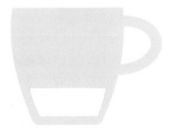

Add a quarter spoon of turmeric powder into the cup. This is about 1 gram of turmeric powder. Turmeric powder is easily available in all grocery and super stores.

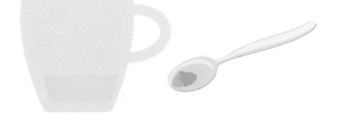

Once you have added the turmeric powder to the milk, place the cup with the milk into a microwave and heat for two minutes. Please keep an eye on the milk. Stop the microwave when the milk rises to prevent it from boiling over. Ideally, this cycle of boiling should be repeated twice to cook the turmeric.

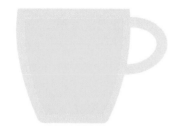

Add some more warm milk. For taste, you can add sugar, syrup or sweetener. Your drink is now ready. Drink this about an hour before you sleep. That should help with the anti-inflammatory effect. You can drink this three times a day, i.e. at breakfast, lunch and in the evening.

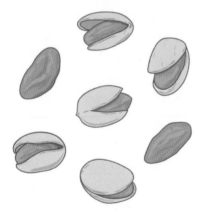

If you are not allergic to pistachio nuts you can take seven to ten kernels of Pistachio nuts with the turmeric latte. Pistachio has melatonin which is the sleep hormone. This should enhance your ability to sleep.

Chapter 10 – The Microbiome (Gut Bacteria)

Introduction
The human intestine contains tens of trillions of individual bacteria known collectively as the "microbiome". It was initially assumed that these bacteria in the gut were just making a few vitamins for us, but research has shown that we gain a lot of benefits from these millions of tiny friends that we have. The levels of gut bacteria a person has can change from the minute they are born. A natural birth through the birth canal exposes infants to a host of micro-organisms that contribute to the quantity of bacteria in the gut [1]. A newborn birthed by a caesarean will not have encountered these micro-organisms and will therefore not have the same levels of gut bacteria. These early bacteria alter the environment within the gut, paving the way for other bacteria to colonize it. This early exposure is, therefore, vital for the overall development of the microbiome (gut bacteria) [1]. Early life feeding also affects gut bacteria. Natural breast milk contains over 600 different species of beneficial bacteria, which help the colonization of the microbiome in the gut. Formula milk does not have the same bacteria and is, therefore, less valuable [1].

How does it work?
Both good and harmful bacteria are contained within the intestine. During digestion, food is broken down and the nutrients are absorbed through the intestinal wall. The intestinal wall also serves another purpose: it prevents unwanted harmful or "bad" bacteria from entering our system. However, the intestine cannot do this alone and needs the help of good bacteria. The good bacteria are constantly multiplying to outnumber the harmful bacteria and prevent them from growing excessively. Unfortunately, when there aren't enough good bacteria, the levels of harmful bacteria rise. The intestinal wall may then "leak" and allow the harmful bacteria to enter our system. The harmful bacteria may not directly cause diseases but can trigger needless immune responses, increasing inflammation in the body.

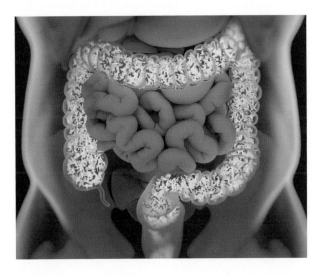

How the microbiome changes (dysbiosis)
Gut bacteria levels and composition can change with age. At around three years, an infant's microbiome has evolved to resemble that of an adult and will remain largely unchanged until they reach old age, where it will begin to decline [1]. Such changes in the microbiome are called gut dysbiosis. Dysbiosis refers to any change in the gut bacteria's composition, whether that is an increase or decrease of any particular category/type of bacteria. Unfortunately, it is unknown if these changes are a cause or consequence of ageing [2]. What is known, though, is that gut bacteria have a strong impact on health, and alterations to bacterial

diversity and functionality are associated with various inflammatory conditions and multiple other disorders [2].

Whilst gut bacteria can affect our health; our diet affects the gut bacteria. This is evident in older people living in residential care. A study by Claesson and colleagues investigated the links between diet, environment, health and gut bacteria in 178 older people [1]. The study found that adults in long- or short-term residential care had lower gut bacteria diversity than those who live in the community, meaning they had fewer types of bacteria within their gut [1]. The researchers observed that 98% of the community dwellers had a high-fibre diet. Conversely, 83% of the participants staying in long-term residential care had low fibre diets. This difference in fibre consumption is thought to be the reason for the disparity in the gut bacteria between the two populations [1]. Such findings hint at the effects diet can have on the microbiome.

What are the effects of changes in the microbiome (gut dysbiosis)?

On the elderly
Changes in gut bacteria (gut dysbiosis) can affect the health of the elderly. For instance, associations have been found between reduced gut bacteria diversity and decreased functional independence [1]. As previously stated, older adults living in long-stay care have a less diverse microbiome than those in the community. The study by Claesson and team concluded that this loss of "community-associated" bacteria is associated with increased frailty and reduced muscle mass (sarcopenia) [1].

Arthritis
Arthritis has also been associated with changes in gut bacteria. It has even been suggested that the microbiome may play a causal role in the development of musculoskeletal diseases [3]. Previous research using animal studies indicated that gut bacteria influenced joint inflammation [3]. Unfortunately, this has not been fully investigated in human patients. However, it has been found that patients with rheumatoid arthritis (RA) and osteoarthritis (OA) have significant differences in the gut and oral bacteria when compared to healthy individuals [3]. Additionally, these alterations in the microbiome resemble the differences found in the gut of patients with other systemic inflammatory conditions, including inflammatory bowel disease and psoriasis [3]. Such findings display a relationship between changes in the gut bacteria (dysbiosis), inflammation and inflammatory diseases. Furthermore, Lorenzo and colleagues reviewed the relevant literature and found that patients with rheumatoid arthritis have higher concentrations of the gut bacteria prevotella copri than people without the condition [3]. The writers concluded that oral and gut dysbiosis seems to play an important role in the cause and development of both rheumatoid and osteoarthritis [3].

Obesity
The gut bacteria are also involved in the regulation of metabolism [4]. It can therefore be assumed that it influences body mass index, weight-management and obesity. Obesity is a global health concern affecting more than 600 million people

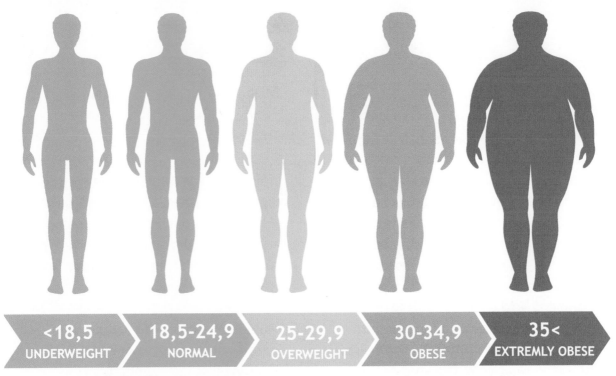

| <18,5 UNDERWEIGHT | 18,5-24,9 NORMAL | 25-29,9 OVERWEIGHT | 30-34,9 OBESE | 35< EXTREMLY OBESE |

Body Mass Index (BMI) = Weight in kgs / (Height in Meters²)

worldwide in 2014 [4]. A study by Ley and team showed that bacteroidetes are decreased in obese people compared to lean people. This loss is reversed with weight loss [4]. These findings reveal that obesity and weight loss are associated with changes in gut bacteria (dysbiosis) [4].

Colorectal cancer (CRC)
Of all the cancers, colorectal cancer is the fourth greatest cause of death worldwide [4]. Like other cancers, colorectal cancer is associated with both genetic and environmental factors, including diet and lifestyle [4]. Moreover, recent research has suggested that the gut microbiome may also play a role in the development of the condition. For example, a study by Wang in 2012 examined faeces of both colorectal cancer patients and healthy patients in order to observe any differences in the faecal bacterial diversity [4]. Patients with colorectal cancer were found to have

significantly higher levels of bacteroides fragilis, a certain form of bacteria within the gut [4].

How can we keep the microbiome healthy and prevent gut dysbiosis?

Diet
There are possible ways to increase the microbiome. Recent research has discovered that changes in diet can affect gut bacteria in both good and bad ways. These changes can consequently affect the immune system and metabolism, as well as body weight and mood. Research published in the Scientific Journal Nature suggests that the gut's microbiome can be altered by diet in just a matter of days [5].

Fermented foods
Fermented foods have also been found to improve the levels of bacteria in the gut. A review in 2018 examined the available

| Aged cheese | Bitter chocolate | Kefir | Sour cream | Miso soup | Pickles | Probiotic milk | Yogurt |

Probiotics - food that contains good bacteria

literature and investigated the effects of fermented foods, including cultured dairy products, fermented sausages, fermented vegetables, soy-fermented foods, and fermented cereal products. The study stated that these products contain high levels of lactic acid bacteria. This form of bacteria has been shown to have health benefits, including the potential to control cholesterol and cancers. The study concluded that fermented food's may provide many essential micronutrients to the gut [6].

Probiotics and prebiotics

Probiotics are live, non-pathogenic microorganisms that provide health benefits when administered in appropriate amounts [6]. Such organisms are a normal part of a healthy human gut microbiome, and their introduction from an external source may benefit the gut. Probiotics can be consumed by eating raw vegetables and fruit, dairy products, and fermented pickles [7]. A literature review by Markowiak and team found various scientific reports which support the use of probiotics, with research indicating that they may be helpful with regard to irritable bowel syndrome, Type II diabetes and bacterial infections [7]. Additionally, probiotics can prevent illness and have been found to contain anti-inflammatory properties [6].

Prebiotics are non-digestible food ingredients that probiotics feed off, enabling a surge in good bacteria populations [6]. Like probiotics, they have been shown to be beneficial for the immune system whilst also having anti-inflammatory effects [6]. When probiotics and prebiotics are used in combination, they become synbiotics, where they can be utilized to promote better gut and overall health [6]. The resulting changes to the gut can help restore or maintain a diverse and functional microbiome. However, the available evidence on this topic is not substantial enough to draw significant conclusions regarding the foods ability to prevent age-related illnesses [6]. Furthermore, it is recommended that probiotics are not used in critically ill patients or patients with weakened immune systems.

| Onion | Soy bean | Asparagus | Bananas | Leek | Bread | Artichoke | Garlic |

Prebiotics - food that feeds the good bacteria

What can be done?
The following foods have been shown to promote better gut health. These can be included in a diet to reap the potential benefits of a healthy microbiome:

- Yoghurts with live cultures
- Sourdough
- Almonds
- Olive oil
- Kefir and other fermented foods

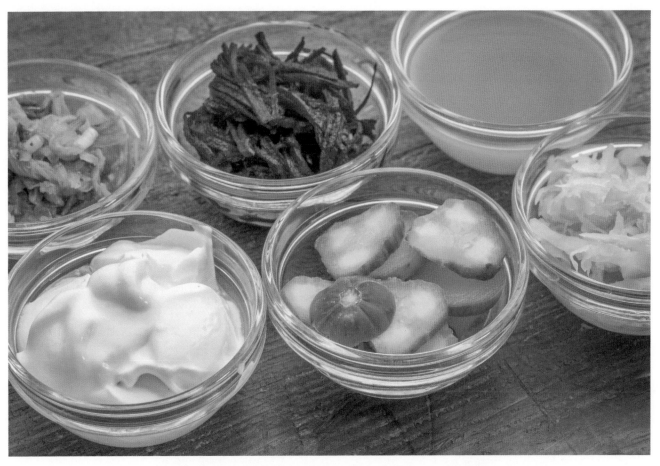

Fermented foods for gut health; kimchi, red beets,
apple cider vinegar, coconut milk yoghurt, cucumber pickles, sauerkraut

Chapter 11 – Rest and Relaxation

Introduction

The greatest form of rest and relaxation (R&R) is sleep, during which we are almost entirely absent of arousal, and our bodies and minds can recharge.

Why sleep?

Sleep is essential for life and health. It plays a vital role in maximising the function of the brain, the immune system, the hormonal system, the cardiovascular system, metabolism and appetite [1]. Research has identified that both the depth and length of sleep are crucial. Normal, healthy sleep is characterized by good quality sleep for seven hours, at an appropriate and regular time, without sleep disturbances and disorders [1]. Shockingly, and despite the importance of sleep, up to 45 million people in Europe have a chronic sleep disorder that affects daily functioning and health [1].

The stages of sleep

There are four stages of sleep, which are repeated various times throughout the night. The completion of all four stages is called a sleep cycle, and each cycle lasts about 90-120 minutes. This cycle is repeated four to five times each night. In a cycle, non-rapid eye movement (NREM) sleep accounts for the first three stages, making up as much as 80% of the time asleep. The first of these stages lasts around five to ten minutes and is the "dozing off" stage, where the body is not yet entirely relaxed. It is easy to be woken during this stage, but if a person is left undisturbed, they swiftly transition to stage two. The second stage starts when the muscles relax, eye movements stop, breathing, heart rate and brainwaves slow, and body temperature drops. This period of light sleep, which lasts around 10-25 minutes, prepares your body for deep sleep. The third stage is deep sleep, where brain waves slow further, and muscle activity stops entirely. It is difficult to be woken when in this stage of sleep, which lasts around 20-40 minutes. During this final stage of NREM sleep, the body releases the growth hormone to build bone and muscle, strengthen its immune system and repair tissues.

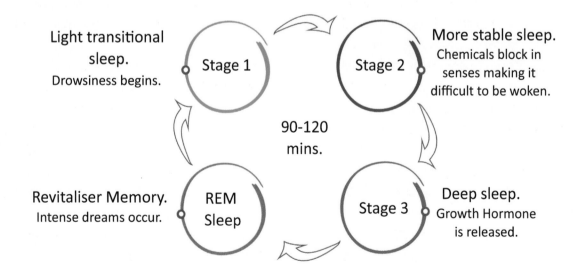

Sleep Cycle stages - the same cycle is repeated many times during the night

However, humans do not dream when in any of the NREM sleep stages. It is during the fourth stage of sleep, known as Rapid Eye Movement sleep (REM), in which dreams occur. During this stage, brain activity increases, but the body is put in a state of near-paralysis (muscle atonia – weakness of muscles), where only the eyes are allowed to move in response to the dreams. Hence the name Rapid Eye Movement sleep. This is an evolutionary adaptation that prevents the limbs from acting out, with the aim of avoiding injury. During this stage of sleep, breathing rate and heart rate quicken, and blood pressure increases. It is also thought that emotion and memories are processed and stored during REM sleep. In the first sleep cycle of the night, REM sleep will last around 10 minutes. With each sleep cycle thereafter, the REM period increases in length. In all, REM sleep makes up around 20% of sleep in adults.

Hormones involved in sleep

1. **Somatotropin**
    The growth hormone somatotropin is intermittently released during sleep, with levels peaking immediately after sleep onset [2]. This hormone stimulates growth, cell reproduction and cell regeneration and is vital to everyday life. Patients with PTSD who struggle to sleep at night exhibit lower growth hormone levels compared to healthy people [2].

2. **Cortisol**
    Cortisol is the stress hormone that regulates motivation, mood and fear. It is tied to the circadian rhythm – the natural and automatic mechanism which regulates the sleep-wake cycle every 24 hours. Cortisol levels increase overnight during sleep and peak in the early morning [2]. This peak stimulates wakefulness in the mornings and contributes to alertness throughout the day. As the day progresses, cortisol levels decrease to aid in bringing about sleep in the evening.

3. **Melatonin**
    Melatonin is the sleep hormone produced by the pineal gland within the brain. Melatonin levels are higher during the night than during the day, with the body only producing it after dark. Watching television, bright lights or reading e-mails late into the night prevents the secretion of melatonin and may disturb sleep [2].

Health consequences of sleep disruption

Short-term psychosocial issues
1. Examples of psychosocial issues include emotional distress and mood disorders, as well as memory and cognitive performance deficits [1]. One study asked the mothers of children treated for leukaemia to report their sleep disruption and their consequent feelings and emotions. These parents often experienced sleep disruption because their child needed care during the night or simply worried about their child's illness. The mothers reported being irritable, impatient and less productive than before their child became ill [1].

2. Sleep disruption is also linked to depression. A 2014 study asked

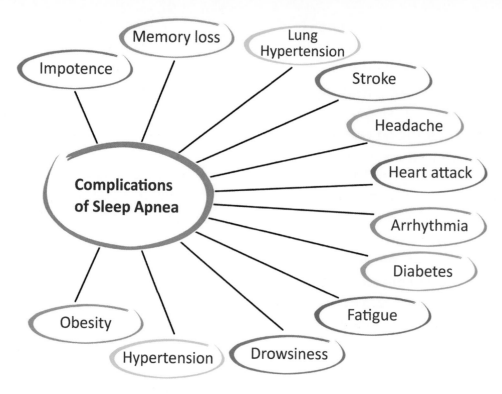

Complications of disturbed sleep

participants to report their sleep quality and required them to complete the Personality Assessment Inventory. Self-reports of sleep disruption were heavily related with symptoms of depression and anxiety [1]. Furthermore, the frequency of the sleep disturbance positively correlated with the severity of the symptoms, meaning the worse the sleep disruption, the worse the depression/anxiety [1].

3. Sleep disruption also alters cognitive performance in various ways, including forming memories, decision-making, risk-taking behaviour and judgement [1]. One study investigated the effects of sleep disruption on daytime functioning. The study showed that disruption to sleep results in reduced ability to process information, impaired attention and decreased motor control [1].

Long-term effects of sleep disruption

1. **Cardiovascular disease**
   Sleep deprivation can cause increased sympathetic nervous system activity, which is responsible for all things related to the fight-or-flight response. As part of the fight-or-flight response, it produces hormones to raise the body's heart rate and awareness and sends extra blood to the muscles, all with the aim of improving the response to danger. As sleep disruption can increase the activity of the sympathetic nervous system, adults who experience sleep disruption can have elevated blood pressure [1]. In another study, difficulty falling asleep, difficulty staying asleep and tiredness when waking were related to heart attacks and high blood pressure [1].

2. Cancer

Sleep deprivation has been shown to accelerate tumour formation and increase cancer risk [1]. In the modern-day, exposure to a lot of light before going to bed is common through watching TVs and looking at mobile phones. However, this unnatural light might confuse the body's sleep system and reduce the amount of melatonin produced. This may lead to the excessive production of reproductive hormones (which melatonin usually suppresses), thus increasing the risk of cancer. Other effects of melatonin also may be diminished. Melatonin has been shown to repair DNA and prevent tumour growth, but both these effects may be reduced by artificial light at night [1].

Furthermore, working shifts during thenight, and therefore having a. disrupted sleeping pattern, has been associated with an increased risk of cancer [1]. In the Nurses' Health Study, the incidence of colorectal cancer was compared in women who never worked night shifts with nurses who worked over 15 years on both day and night shifts. The study showed that the night-shift nurses were 1.3 times more likely to develop colorectal cancer [1].

3. Metabollic Disorders

Disrupted sleep has been associated with weight gain and other weight-related issues in adults [1]. A five-year study measured sleep over several nights using wrist actigraphy – a wristwatch-like tool that measures rest and activity cycles. The researchers then observed any relationships between sleep duration/disruption and body mass index (BMI) at a six-year follow-up. The results showed that greater fragmentation of sleep was strongly associated with increases in BMI [1]. Sleep disruption may also alter blood glucose control [1]. Blood glucose levels are maintained at a steady-state by hormones like insulin. One study identified that sleep disruption resulted in decreased insulin sensitivity. Insulin sensitivity refers to the responsiveness of various cells in the body to insulin. High insulin sensitivity enables the body to use glucose more effectively and thereby reduce blood sugar levels. Sleep disruption thus decreases insulin sensitivity and increases the risk of diabetes [1]. Four further large studies also showed that sleep disruption was associated with an 84% greater relative risk of developing Type II diabetes [1].

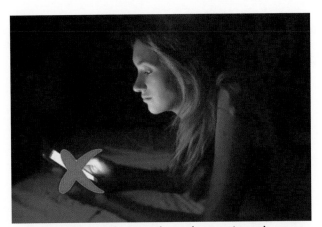

Going through emails or browsing the net or social media at night or just before sleep prevents restful sleep. Avoid bright screens for 90 minutes before sleep time

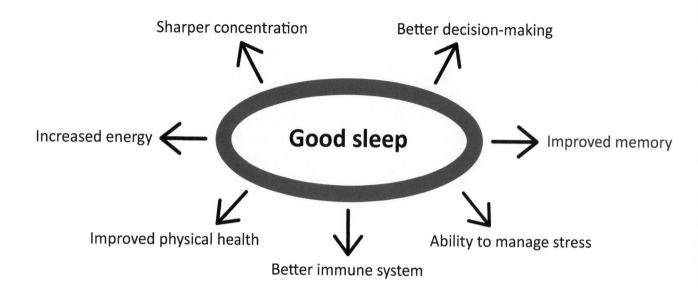

Sharper concentration

Better decision-making

Increased energy

Good sleep

Improved memory

Improved physical health

Better immune system

Ability to manage stress

What are the benefits of sleep?
Aside from the reduced risk of the conditions outlined previously, good quality, regular sleep can have multiple benefits. These include:

1. **Memory**
    Sleep allows the retention of short-term memories by converting them into long-term memories
    This is thought to happen in the third stage of sleep (NREM), also known as short-wave sleep [3].
2. **Physical functions**
    During exercise and typical day-to-day activity, muscles become damaged (this is completely normal) and must repair themselves to become stronger. Sleep can accommodate and facilitate this healing. It is, therefore, vital that one has a sufficient amount of sleep every night [4].

What can be done – How can I sleep better?

Reduce exposure to blue light.
Before discovering electricity, nights were dark and provided the ideal condition to rest and sleep. However, in modern times, sleeping when the sun has gone down is not essential as artificial bright lights can be created. With the invention of the television and the mobile phone, humans are exposed to brighter, blue light late into the evening. This is often the case right before sleep when people scroll through social media or watch their favourite TV shows. Blue light suppresses melatonin production and causes neurophysiological arousal [5]. In other words, it prevents rest and relaxation. It is therefore recommended that for at least an hour before bed, individuals read a book or newspaper in order to reduce the

effect that blue light can have on sleep. Allowing this break from screens will improve sleep quality and duration.

A study on insomniacs compared the use of amber lenses that block the blue light versus clear lenses. The use of amber lenses for two hours prior to bedtime for seven consecutive days provided improved quality and length of sleep. The same study also showed how blocking the blue light with amber-tinted lenses improved quality of life and decreased distress in the study subjects [5].

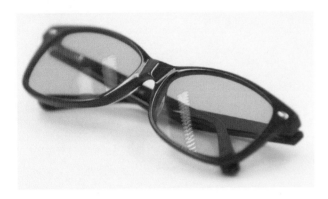

Exercise

Physical exercise and activity promote sleep quantity and quality. A study in 2008 found that sleep improved both in quality and quantity in women who were physically active as compared to those who were sedentary [6]. However, strenuous exercise should stop two to three hours prior to bedtime.

Regularity

Maintaining a regular sleeping pattern will safeguard the body's natural body clock. Therefore, going to bed at the same time each evening and waking after the recommended amount of time each day ensures that sleep remains good quality. Similar to how we may have an alarm to wake us up, it may be equally important to have an alarm to go to bed.

Pistachios

Pistachio nuts have been found to contain melatonin – the chemical which helps regulate the body's biological sleep cycle. Hence, the consumption of pistachios is recommended for those who do not sleep well, as the melatonin within should aid in promoting good sleep. It is recommended that these nuts are taken as a snack about 90 minutes before bedtime.

During normal sleep, blood pressure (BP) usually decreases (dips) in what is known as "nocturnal dipping". Sleep disorders can reduce this physiological change and increase the risk of high blood pressure. As a result, patients who do not exhibit these dips in blood pressure are up to 66% more likely to experience a cardiovascular event [7]. Pistachios have been found to increase this dip in blood pressure, thus reducing such risks. Sauder and team investigated this in their 2014 study. 30 adult participants, aged 40 to 74 years,

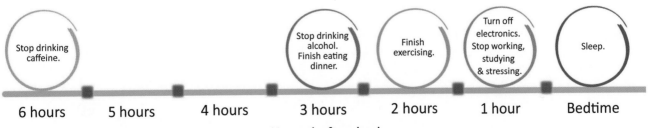

| 6 hours | 5 hours | 4 hours | 3 hours | 2 hours | 1 hour | Bedtime |

Stop drinking caffeine.

Stop drinking alcohol. Finish eating dinner.

Finish exercising.

Turn off electronics. Stop working, studying & stressing.

Sleep.

Hours before bed

The perfect night's sleep starts before you get into bed.

consumed a moderate-fat diet containing high levels of pistachios for four weeks. The researchers found that blood pressure was significantly decreased following the diet, with the largest reductions observed during sleep [7]. The benefits of pistachios are, therefore, two-fold. Not only can they reduce blood pressure during sleep, but they can also improve the quality of sleep overall.

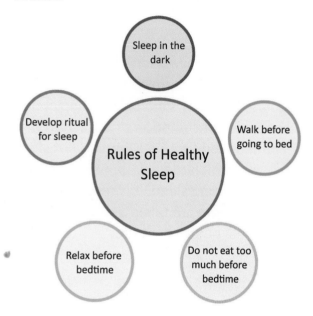

Chapter 12 – Family and Friends

Introduction

Family and friends play an essential role in dealing with life's challenges. They provide support and encouragement when needed most, helping shape an individual's well-being throughout their lifetime. Aesop's fable of the lion and the mouse allows us to understand why such relationships are essential and how simple acts of support and kindness can go a long way.

A lion lay deep asleep, with his huge head resting on his paws. As he slept, a small, timid mouse came upon him suddenly. The sight of the lion shocked the mouse, and in her fright and haste to get away, she ran across the lion's nose. The lion stirred and awoke from his slumber. Angry that his sleep was disturbed, he laid his huge paw on the tiny creature to kill her. The poor mouse begged the lion to spare her life and promised to repay him someday. The lion was amused to think that a tiny mouse could ever help him, but he was generous and let the mouse go.

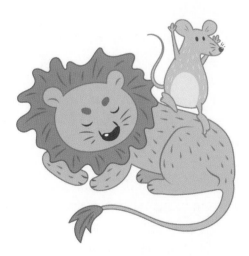

Sometime later, the lion was stalking his prey through the forest when he became caught in a hunter's net. Unable to free himself, the lion roared in frustration. Somewhere in the distance, the mouse heard and recognised the roar and rushed off to find him. Before long, she found him struggling in the net. The mouse immediately began gnawing at the rope until she cut through the ties that bound the lion. The lion was soon free and very grateful that he had not killed the mouse when she woke him. "You were amused when I said I would repay you," said the mouse. "Now you can see that even a mouse can help a lion." [1]

Through kindness and empathy, the lion let the mouse live when she stumbled upon him. In his time of need, the mouse repaid the lion with the same kindness and empathy he had shown her. The story shows that an act of kindness is never wasted and that even relationships formed in the most unlikely of circumstances can provide benefits for those involved.

What is family?

What makes a family is subjective. A "traditional" western family would consist of a husband and wife alongside their child/children. This is called a nuclear family and is commonplace in the western world. In nuclear families, the children usually move away from their parental home once they become adults. Conversely, in many cultures worldwide, children stay in the family home, providing for their parents and grandparents throughout adulthood. This is what is known as a joint family. Up to four generations can live under the same roof in a joint family, supporting and caring for one another. These different variations of family show that no one definition can truly explain what family is. The construct is culturally dependent, and the definition may change depending on the local traditions and ideals. A recent description states that family is: "People related by marriage, birth, consanguinity or legal adoption, who share a common kitchen and financial resources regularly" [2].

This definition, however, is more suited to cultures in which joint families are common and not those where nuclear families are the norm. Children from nuclear families, who fly the nest, would scarcely believe that they are no longer a family member just because they are financially independent or have their own home. A more fitting, universal definition would state that family is "people related by marriage,birth, consanguinity or legal adoption, who emotionally support and

care for one another regularly".

Family relationships play a central role in shaping and maintaining a person's well-being throughout life [3]. Given the ever-ageing population, these relationships are becoming even more critical to well-being. Older people now require more care in later life [3]. They may also rely on their family relationships for support, as their ties with people from other social domains (i.e., workplace) decrease over time [3]. These factors reveal the need to understand better the effects family relationships have on well-being and health, especially in later life.

What are friends?
"You can't choose your family, but you can choose your friends" is a very old phrase that often rings true. The closest of friends will be there through the hardest parts of life, such as illness or personal tragedy. We may often know our friends better than our own

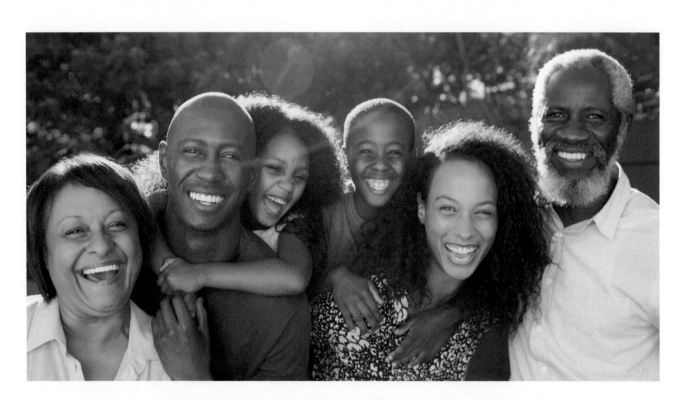

family. Whether or not such friends can be family is up to personal and cultural interpretation.

Humans are naturally social [4]. As a result, friendship is part of everyday human life. Friendship is so vital that severing bonds with friends can cause health problems and depression. Additionally, social exclusion can result in feelings similar to physical pain [5].

Social relationships – on the decrease?

Social relationships are any relationships, whether that is with family or friends. Three major components consistently evaluate them. These include:

1. How much the relationship plays a role in an individual's overall social life [4].
2. How often the people in the relationship meet and interact with one another in a supportive way (i.e., received social support) [4].
3. The person's beliefs and perceptions about the available support from the people in their social relationships (i.e., perceived social support) [4].

Having a strong network of family and friends (social relationships) can have many health benefits. Researchers have previously theorised that social relationships improve health by providing resources (e.g. knowledge and emotional support) that help to deal with life's stressors (e.g. illness, life events etc.) [4]. Another theory is that social relationships may directly encourage healthy behaviours. For instance, being part of a social network increases a person's conformity to health care norms and self-

care [4]. Furthermore, being members of a social network provides individuals with meaningful roles, which increase self-esteem and purpose in life [4].

Although humans are social animals, the modern way of life significantly reduces the quantity and quality of social relationships. As previously stated, people no longer choose to live in extended families. Individuals now choose to move away from their parents, going as far as the other side of the world. Many now also delay having children or getting married [4].

Besides, people are now obsessed with social media, including platforms like Facebook and Instagram. Individuals can have thousands of "friends" on these websites, many of whom they may have not even met. Although they are referred to as friends, if Facebook relationships were assessed using the three components outlined previously, they would not fulfil the definition of a social relationship.

Social media relationships are not supportive or even truly interactive. Nor can individuals really trust every social media contact they have, as they would their closest friends. Only perhaps a

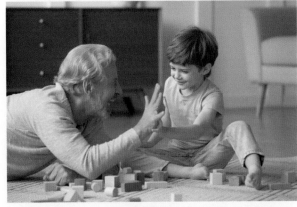

Relationships that mutually benefit both

handful (five or six) of an individual's thousand social media followers would actually be classed as friends. Moreover, people's interpretation of what friendship actually entails is being clouded by social media. Individuals attempt to impress total strangers with an exaggerated portrayal of their life by posting pictures or anecdotes on their profiles. People worry excessively about how they present themselves and how they look to other social media users (many of whom are strangers) whilst not receiving the care and support that is usually provided by real-life friendships.

Consequently, social media relationships rarely help with life's stresses. In fact, they can make them worse. As a result of this, the use of social media is linked to depression and anxiety. A study by Shensa and the team asked 1,730 adults aged 19 to 32 to complete an online survey, where they reported their social media use and their symptoms of anxiety and depression (if any). They found that people who use social media most frequently and for long periods were significantly more likely to show symptoms of anxiety and depression than people who never/rarely use social media [6].

As a consequence of these factors combined, loneliness is becoming more and more common. In a survey by the Mental Health Foundation, 10% of people in the UK reported often feeling lonely [4]. 33% of the people surveyed said they have a close friend or relative who they think is extremely lonely, whilst 50% believe that people are getting lonelier in general [4]. These statistics suggest that the modern way of life, where joint families are less common, is resulting in increased loneliness and higher depression and anxiety rates. This may have a severe negative impact on both the physical and mental health of affected individuals.

What are the benefits of family and friends?

Benefits of having children
Despite what people may think, given the stress involved, having children can increase longevity. A nationwide study in Sweden contained all Swedish men and women born between 1911 and 1925 and their children, who were all followed over time [7]. The researchers calculated the age-specific deaths each calendar year for both individuals with children and individuals without children. They then compared the results. The researchers found that men who had children lived an average of two years longer than men who didn't have children, whilst women with children lived 1.5 years longer than women with no children [7].

Benefits of adopting children
Adopting children can also have positive effects on health. One study in 2018 investigated this by observing Swedish register data and studying the mortality

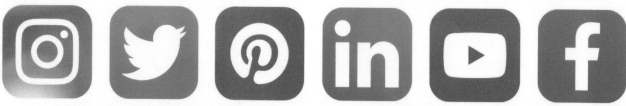

Are they real social relationships that we can depend on in a time of need?

rates among parents who adopted their children but had no biological children [8]. Mothers who adopted one child increased their life expectancy by three years compared to women without children [8]. The researchers also compared adoptive parent mortality rates to those who had biological children. The results showed that the relative risk of death was always lower for adoptive parents than biological parents, indicating that adopting children has a greater impact on longevity [8]. The study also stated that mortality rates were even lower for parents who adopted more than one child [8]. For example, adoptive mothers with two or more children lived five years longer, on average, than women who did not adopt or have any child [8].

Benefits of family relationships

Thomas and team conducted a review of the evidence for family relationships and well-being. Being happily married was associated with better mental and physical health. The strength of the health benefits from marriage was comparable to the benefit that giving up smoking or decreasing obesity can have on well-being [3]. Adult children who care for their parents or grandparents experience benefits to their own health, as providing emotional support and care are associated with better well-being [3]. Furthermore, grandparents and grandchildren who have good relationships with one another also have higher well-being [3]. The majority of grandparents engage in meaningful activities with their grandchildren and feel close to them.

Benefits of social relationships

A review by Holt-Lunstad and colleagues looked into the effects social relationships can have on mortality. The review included 148 studies, including over 300,000 participants. Results indicated that participants with stronger social relationships had a 50% reduced risk of death [4]. These results remained consistent when factoring in age, sex, initial health status and cause of death [4]. The researchers concluded that having strong social relationships can reduce mortality, similar to how well-established risk factors increase it (e.g., smoking, obesity) [4].

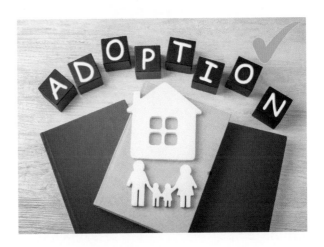

Lessons from Okinawa

In the Blue Zone "Okinawa", where people live longer than elsewhere in the world, residents work hard to maintain solid, close friendships. Okinawans commonly belong to a "moais" – a group of five friends who are committed to each other for life from around the age of five. The tradition of membership in one of these groups ensures secure social networks [9]. They provide financial and emotional support and relieve stress [9]. Friends in these groups meet every day, without fail, to share stories and beverages. If one friend does not attend at the usual time of the meeting, the other four will walk to their house to check on them [9].

Okinawans attribute their longevity to these social networks, suggesting that such friendships are vital to living a long and happy life.

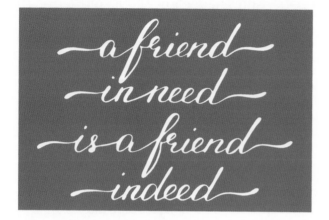

How to improve social networks/relationships

"Moais"

Creating a "moais" with close friends and committing to meeting once a week, perhaps for a coffee morning or lunch, can provide many health benefits. For example, having friendship groups as committed as the ones seen in Okinawa may increase longevity.

Increased interaction with family

Even if living as nuclear families, it is important to increase the interaction between grandchildren and grandparents. These interactions can provide increased emotional support and social nurturing in a safe environment.

University of the 3ʳᵈ Age (U3A)

The U3A is an international organisation that allows older people to meet regularly to share knowledge and skills. Membership is restricted to retirees and provides a welcoming environment where they attend classes run by other members. For instance, retired music teachers can provide piano lessons for the rest of the group. Membership in this organisation can act like a "moais", providing the foundations for friendships and social support. Research has found that U3A attendees have better general health and higher satisfaction in life than those who do not belong to such an organisation.

Religion

Belonging to a religious group can also help provide support networks and friendship groups. People with similar interests and values are connected through their religious groups. These people then become members of strong support networks, further improving their social network and social interactions.

What can be done?

In our later years, options may be limited to extend our families. However, there is still a lot we can do in the wider community, whether it may be looking after grandchildren or helping other children in difficulty. For instance, temporarily fostering children in need for a few years provides adults with an opportunity to enlarge their families and gain the associated health benefits. Not only will the adults benefit, but so do the children who may desperately require safe and reliable housing. You could also spend more time with your friends and devote time to making new friends – whether that is through a social group, neighbours, or even through existing friends. The joy that can come from widening our social circle and helping children is a very rewarding feeling, so why not make it a priority?

Chapter 13 – Ikigai – Japanese for "Purpose in Life"

Introduction

Purpose in Life (PIL) is described as having goals, a sense of direction and a feeling that there is meaning in existence [1]. Engagement in daily activities which match one's long-term aims is the basis for purposeful living. For instance, hobbies, careers and household tasks can all give an individual a sense of this. However, for the majority of people, finding their purpose in life is not easy. Life in the modern-day is full of distractions, preventing people from discovering their true goals and purpose. Pressures to gloat on social media cause individuals to stray from their innate passions and values. People instead focus on portraying an altered version of reality to give the impression of a "perfect life". Additionally, societal pressures to earn more money and be more professionally successful mean many people focus on these aspects of life rather than what makes them happy.

Consider this story…

Patrick is a successful man: he is the director of a large financial company. He earns an excellent salary, has a lovely wife and two children aged ten and nine. They all live in a large house in a nice suburb. By all standards, Patrick appears to be living a fulfilling life. However, this is not the case. Patrick actually feels unhappy and empty with his current existence. He has little purpose in life. One day, his wife falls pregnant. He and his wife are elated with this surprise addition. Nine months go by and a baby daughter is born. However, the baby is born with learning difficulties, which devastates Patrick and his wife. They feel that this is a terrible situation of bad luck and are extremely upset. As time passes, Patrick begins to realise that this baby is giving him a purpose. The baby's constant calls for attention and love provide Patrick with reasons to live for. Each morning, he goes to work with the needs of his baby in mind. It prompts him to work harder to ensure the safety of her future. Patrick realises just how empty his life was before his baby and considers

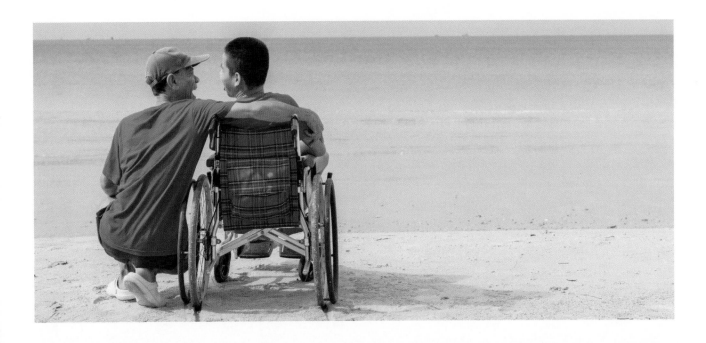

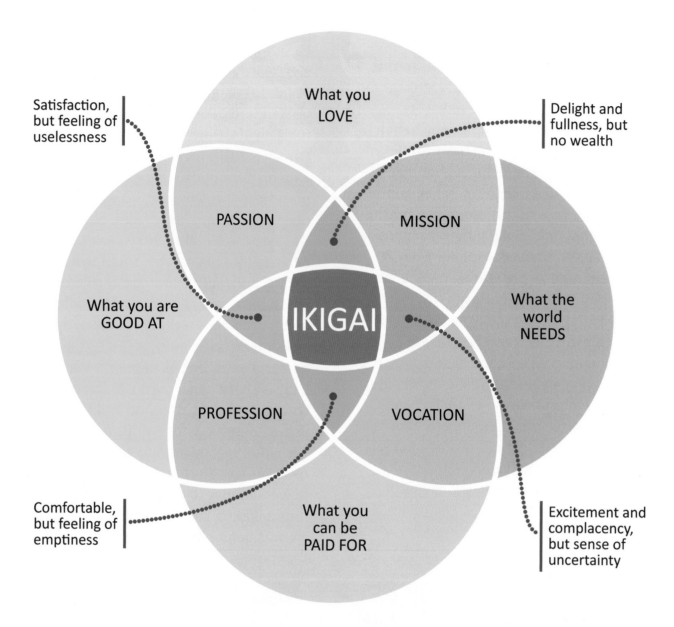

Satisfaction,
but feeling of
uselessness

Delight and
fullness, but
no wealth

What you
LOVE

PASSION

MISSION

What you are
GOOD AT

IKIGAI

What the
world
NEEDS

PROFESSION

VOCATION

Comfortable,
but feeling of
emptiness

What you
can be
PAID FOR

Excitement and
complacency,
but sense of
uncertainty

what it would be like without her. He determines that his life is better for having her in it and that it is worth living because of her existence. This story demonstrates that, no matter how successful an individual is, this may not provide satisfaction and fulfilment. In most corporate jobs, you are striving to achieve the goal of your employer. Studies have shown that having a purpose, where goals are self-endorsed, is a significant contributor to good well-being and health.

Therefore, it is vital that, especially in later life, people continue to seek tasks and goals that make them feel fulfilled.

"Ikigai" – What is it?
"Ikigai" is a Japanese concept that has been translated to mean "life worth living" [2]. The word compounds two Japanese phrases: "iki" (to live) and "gai" (reason) [3]. It describes a certain state of psychological well-being, where an individual has a direction in life and a

motivation for living (purpose) [2]. In Japan's most recognized dictionary, "ikigai" is defined as "joy and a sense of well-being from being alive" and also of "realizing the value of being alive" [2].

Everyone has "ikigai". The task is to find and nurture it, as it will bring a profound sense of fulfilment. This is believed to make a person's existence meaningful and worthwhile. In the western world, it is not uncommon for people to struggle to get out of bed in the morning. The presence of "ikigai" reduces the occurrence of this in Japanese culture.

Author Dan Buettner, who wrote the book *Blue Zones: Lessons for Living Longer from the People Who've Lived the Longest*, suggested that "ikigai" may be one of the reasons why people from Okinawa, Japan live longer than people elsewhere. Buettner states that Okinawans have less desire to retire, as they enjoy their jobs, and will continue to work as long as they remain healthy, helping them retain purpose. Residents here also fulfil their "ikigai" by fishing to feed their families, or by performing martial arts [3].

What are the benefits of "ikigai"?

Psychological well-being

In modern society, stress is common. It can be caused by work, bills, and family problems (to name a few). When humans are stressed, the body releases the hormone cortisol. This hormone suppresses the immune system, meaning the body is less able to recover from injury and illness. Cortisol also increases the risk of heart attack and stroke. Fortunately, having a purpose in life may help as it is correlated with higher resilience. Resilience is defined as the ability to adapt and cope with life's challenges. It has been reported as an important variable in ageing successfully. Resilience helps individuals deal with stress and reduces the occurrence of depression. It also helps people to find a positive life balance and, over time, improves self-perception of health [1].

A study by Sone and team investigated the effects of "ikigai" on the health (including stress) and mortality of over 40,000 Japanese adults [2]. Of the 43,391 participants, 59% indicated that they had a sense of "ikigai", 36.4% were uncertain and

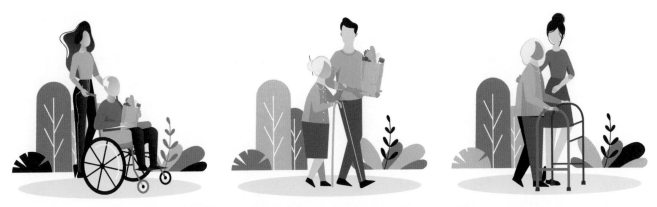

Helping others can provide a purpose in life

4.6% indicated that they had no "ikigai" [2]. The researchers found that only 12% of people who described having "ikigai" reported high levels of mental stress, compared with 36.3% of the people who reported having no "ikigai" [2]. Such results showcase a relationship between purpose in life and reduced stress. Consequently, these findings indicate that the threat of stress-related conditions (stroke etc.) may be reduced by having "ikigai".

Cardiovascular disease (CVD)

One such stress-related condition is cardiovascular disease. Cardiovascular disease is an umbrella term used to describe a range of conditions that affect the blood vessels which are caused by narrowing of the arteries (angina, heart attack, stroke and heart failure). Stress can increase blood pressure and cholesterol and may promote the build-up of plaque within the arteries. All these factors increase the threat of cardiovascular disease. In their study, Sone and colleagues first assessed the participant's sense of "ikigai" by simply asking, "Do you have "ikigai" in your life" [2].

Participants were then required to attend a follow-up seven years later. The researchers then observed any differences in all-cause and specific-cause death rates between those with "ikigai" and those without. The study found that participants who reported that they did not have "ikigai" were three times more likely to die from cardiovascular disease [2]. Stroke was specifically identified and highlighted during the study. A stroke is a condition which causes damage to the brain when the artery to part of the brain is blocked.

The researchers found that participants without "ikigai" were 3.6 times more likely to die of stroke [2]. These results reveal a significant relationship between purpose in life, reduced stress, and decreased incidence of cardiovascular disease.

Alzheimer's disease

Alzheimer's disease is an irreversible brain disorder that progressively destroys thinking and memory skills until affected individuals can no longer complete the simplest of tasks. An investigation into the effects of having purpose on the incidence of Alzheimer's was carried out in 2010. Participants included 900 community-dwelling older adults without dementia who attended a follow-up seven years after the study's onset. Participants' purpose in life was assessed using a questionnaire that asked for responses to statements such as, "I have a sense of direction and purpose in life" and "My daily activities seem trivial and unimportant to me". It was found that people with a high score on the 'purpose in life' measure were approximately 2.4 times more likely to remain free of Alzheimer's [4].

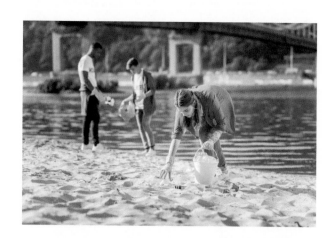

Overall Mortality

All-cause mortality refers to death by any

means. The study by Sone et al. found that, of the 43,391 participants who started the study, 3048 had died by the time of the seven-year follow-up [2]. Although people, both with and without "ikigai", had died within this period, those without purpose were 2.5 times more likely to have passed away [2].

A further study by Hill and Turiano had a similar structure but over 14 years. They found that adults with purpose lived longer than their counterparts during the 14 years of assessment. Interestingly, this reduced mortality was not conditional on retirement status. In other words, purposeful adults who had retired lived just as long as those who had not retired.

Retirement itself is associated with increased health risks, including an enlarged threat of cardiovascular disease [5]. These results show that having a purpose during retirement may prevent these retirement-associated health risks, thus showing the importance of purpose in life. Hill and Turiano also went on to suggest that "healthy ageing" may be influenced by daily physical activity and goal achievement [5]. It should also be noted that people with purpose are more likely to engage in positive health behaviours, such as physical exercise. Subsequently, they will benefit from consistently better health and, in turn, the potential for increased longevity [1].

How do I improve my "ikigai"?
"Ikigai" is seen as the combination of the four elements (see diagram on page 75). What you love; what you are good at; what you can be paid for, and; what the world needs. Ask yourself the following questions

to find your purpose:

1) **What you love (your passion and motivation)**
   a) What would you do if money was not a worry?
   b) What would you enjoy doing over a long weekend or holiday?
   c) What is exciting for you?
   d) What are you enthusiastic about?
2) **What the world needs (your mission)**
   a) What would you like to do to help society?
   b) What social issues emotionally affect you?
   c) Will your work still be relevant in the future?
   d) Will people pay for what you're selling?
3) **What you are good at (your vocation – natural talents)**
   a) What are you best at?
   b) With more training and experience, could you become among the greatest at it?
4) **What you get paid for (your profession – what puts bread on the table)**
   a) Do you get, or have you ever been, paid for what you do?
   b) Are you making a good living? Can you eventually make a good living with the work you do?

The space in the middle of these four elements is where your "ikigai" lies. Let us look at an example to find out Mrs Pradeep's "ikigai". Mrs Pradeep is 66 and retired from the civil service last year. Like many in this position, her circle of friends has suddenly decreased as she does not meet her colleagues from work anymore. She finishes her household chores within a few hours and watches daytime TV and sits in front of a TV from 16:00 to 22:00.

This is not a healthy lifestyle - this is just Mrs Pradeep filling her time. However, she can find her "ikigai" and become fruitful. Let us help her with the diagram on page 68.

What do you love?
Mrs Pradeep loves watching TV, cooking and reading books.

What does the world need?
Mrs Pradeep could become a freelance editor and copy writer. Websites like Fiverr© provide opportunities. Mrs Pradeep could become a professional cook.

What are you good at?
Mrs Pradeep is good both at cooking and document editing.

What do you get paid for?
The pub near Mrs Pradeep advertises for a chef. Mrs Pradeep applies for the job and goes for the interview. She is not successful and does not get the job.
She now advertises herself as a freelance editor on www.fiverr.com. After about a week, she gets her first job. Slowly the freelance editing tasks increase. She is also getting paid for it.

Two years have passed, and she is now very busy though she has retired. She now only watches TV for an hour or two. She is busy with her freelance editing job. She has joined the U3A and is part of a new group of friends. They walk 3 times a week.

In a similar manner you can find your "ikigai". Whatever sits in the middle area is your "ikigai".

Chapter 14 – Faith

Introduction
Consider this story

A young businessman was near bankruptcy. Debt collectors were chasing him, and associates were demanding payment. He could see no way out. Stressed, he sat on a park bench. He recollected his entire life, and images from childhood to the present flashed from memory. At that moment, an elderly man approached and sat down beside him. "I can see something is troubling you", the elderly gentleman said. The businessman began to pour his heart out to the elderly gentleman, describing his difficulties and explaining that there was no apparent way out.

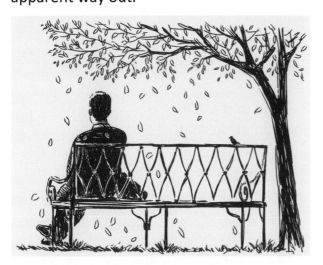

After listening intently, the elderly gentleman said, "I believe I can help you." He drew out a chequebook and asked for the businessman's name. As he wrote out the cheque, the young man peered over his shoulder, seeing a large sum of money being written on it. The old man then placed it into an envelope before sealing it and handing it over. "I'm an old man with too much money; I don't need all of it. Please take this and try to save your business." The young man took the envelope in his hands and stared at it in disbelief. The young businessman was in shock. "My money worries are over", he thought, a wave of relief passing over him. The businessman decided not to tell his family about his encounter with the elderly gentleman or the cheque that he had received. He also did not cash in the cheque but instead locked it up in his safe. Knowing that the cheque was there in reserve, the young man started to rebuild his business. With renewed confidence and optimism, he began building his business by making small deals and renegotiating contracts. Over time, the businessman started doing larger and larger deals. Before long, he was out of debt, and his company was profitable.

It had been a few years since he had received the cheque from the elderly gentleman. During this period, the businessman had not returned to the park nor had any contact with the elderly gentleman. Since he had now turned around his business, he decided to visit the park in the hope that he could thank the elderly unknown friend and return his unused cheque. The young man sat on the same park bench and waited for the elderly gentleman to show up. For a long time, there was no sign of him. Eventually, the elderly gentleman appeared. Immediately, the businessman stood up to greet and thank him. However, before he could finish his greeting and hand the envelope back, a nurse came running over. "I'm so glad I caught him!" she exclaimed. "I hope he hasn't been bothering you. He often escapes from the nursing home and hands out cheques to random people, telling them that he is a wealthy man." The nurse ushered the old man away with her, leaving the businessman alone in disbelief.

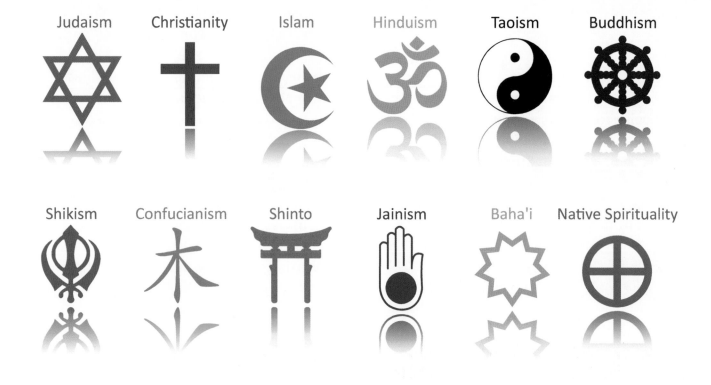

Judaism	Christianity	Islam	Hinduism	Taoism	Buddhism

Shikism	Confucianism	Shinto	Jainism	Baha'i	Native Spirituality

The businessman realized that the cheque, despite being worthless, provided the faith and self-belief needed to give him the power to rescue his business. This story really does show that, with faith, almost anything is possible.

Spirituality and religion

Both the terms "spirituality" and "religion" are interrelated but are separate entities, but both provide positive outcomes in disease and health. Spirituality is practised by an individual and involves a sense of peace and purpose with an understanding of the meaning of life. People who are spiritual believe in an external force but do not necessarily accredit any name to it. Religion, on the other hand, is a specific set of beliefs and customs followed by a group or community. 59% of the world's population describes themselves as religious [1]. Though most of the world's population is religious, it is only very recently that science and medicine have accepted the influence of religion on physical, mental, and emotional health.

Religion and ageing

The human cell has 23 pairs of chromosomes. The chromosomes are made up of genes. The chromosomes and the genes contain all the information for biological survival. At the end of each chromosome are caps called telomeres. They are like the stiff ends of shoelaces. These aglets or the stiff ends in the shoelaces protect the shoelace from fraying. Similarly, the telomeres protect the chromosome from becoming shorter. A part of the ageing process is the reduction in the length of the telomere, with small segments of the ends dropping off. Different factors are involved in this process. Mechanisms which prevent this shortening can decrease ageing and promote youthfulness. A study by Hill and co-workers [2] analysed the telomere length of 1252 adults in Davidson County,

Tennessee, USA. They identified that adults who practised religion and prayed regularly had longer telomere lengths as compared to adults who did not practice religion.

Religion and Alzheimer's disease

Alzheimer's disease is an irreversible degenerative disorder of the brain which affects memory and cognitive ability. As the disease progresses, patients are unable to think, comprehend, plan and problem solve. It mainly affects older people. Autopsy specimen analysis shows the presence of plaques and tangles in the brain of patients who have Alzheimer's disease. The autopsy specimens also show the loss of connections between the different nerve cells. A meta-analysis of 11 studies by Agli and co-workers [3] showed that spirituality and religion seemed to decrease the cognitive decline in Alzheimer's. They suggested some possible mechanisms by which this was possible. Reciting prayers involves memorising and recalling phrases. This improves memory, concentration, attention and repetition. Accomplishing these tasks requires utilising and thereby strengthening frontal neural circuits. In addition to this, putting their lives in the hands of God seemed to decrease anxiety and worry. This made believers more confident of a future than non-believers. Involvement in community prayers also increased social interaction. This increased social interaction provided greater opportunities to share and communicate, which also decreased anxiety and depression. Overall, patients who practised spirituality and religion had slower cognitive decline, improved coping strategies, and a better quality of life.

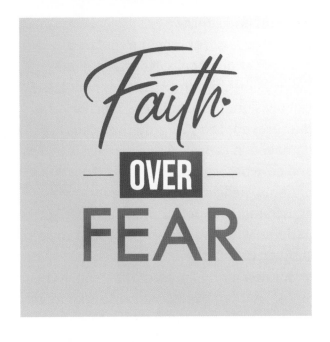

Religion and coronary artery disease

The heart pumps the blood to the various organs and parts of the body. To perform this function, the heart also requires blood supply for its own nutrition and oxygen. The coronary arteries are the arteries within the heart that supply blood to the heart muscle. Blockage of these blood vessels is called coronary artery disease. High blood pressure and diabetes are linked to increased coronary disease. Banerjee and co-workers analysed data from a Canadian survey in Saskatchewan. The sample size was 5442, of which 27.4% attended religious activities more than once a week, 34.9% attended religious activities three to 12 times a year, and 37.7% attended once a year or not at all [4]. Attending weddings and funerals were not included as religious activities. Coronary heart disease, high blood pressure and diabetes were found less in individuals who attended religious activities more than once a week as compared to those who attended once a year or not at all [4].

Religion and cancer

Cancer occurs from the unregulated multiplication of cells. Normal growth involves mechanisms that stop needless cell division. Unfortunately, mechanisms that prevent the overgrowth of cells are damaged in cancer. A meta-analysis by Jim and co-workers looked at data from 32,000 patients. Religion and spirituality were associated with better physical health in patients who had cancer [5]. The study also showed that patients who practise religion or spirituality find greater meaning in their illness and can overcome existential fears [5]. Having faith in an external force provided a greater resilience to withstand the crises. The National Health Interview Survey in the US showed that 69% of patients with cancer participated in prayer as compared to only 45% in the general population.

Religion and chronic pain

Some conditions like fibromyalgia, back pain, migraine, and chronic fatigue are associated with severe pain. Addressing the chronic pain in these conditions can become a challenge. The study by Baetz and co-workers used the Canadian Community Health Survey (2002), which obtained data from 37,000 individuals who were 15 years of age or older. Their data showed that patients who are both religious and spiritual were able to cope with the pain and had better psychological well-being. The authors suggested that increased social connections that result from attending religious services and meetings, better acceptance of illness and the ability to view life from a detached perspective helped religious chronic pain sufferers to cope with their pain better [6].

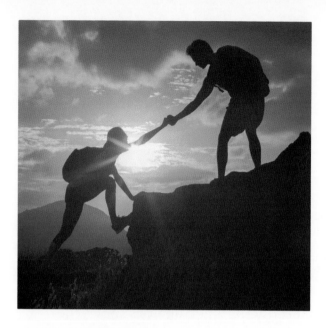

What can you do?

The positive benefits of spirituality and religion may not automatically be achieved by attending religious events regularly. Self-discipline, abstinence from risky and unhelpful behaviour, support and friendship from the community may all form part of the positive benefits of spirituality and religion. Similar to the story at the beginning of this chapter, the faith that a supportive greater force exists provides the optimism and positivity that is required to navigate the difficult valleys of life. We are not inanimate objects, and therefore are affected by emotions and feelings.

You could join a local religious group or go to spiritual workshops to explore faith and to meet like-minded people. Many rehab programs like Alcoholic Anonymous are based on the belief in an external superior force. Similar addiction programs have been very successful.

The Advent health group propose a model for a healthier life and call it **CREATION** [7].

This is a biblical model, based on the Gospel of Matthew, Chapter 11, Verse 28 "Come to me, all you who are weary and burdened, and I will give you rest.". The components of the model form the acronym – CREATION.

Choice – Make positive choices in life.
Rest – Rest to regenerate and recoup
Environment – Space that surrounds you
Activity – Adequate mental and physical activity
Trust – Relationship with God
Interpersonal Relationships – Family and friends
Outlook – Remain positive and optimistic
Nutrition – Good, healthy and wholesome diet.

The website Creation Life (https://www.creationlife.com/) provides useful resources including recipes.

Chapter 15 – Fasting

Introduction
Fasting is defined as the willful abstinence from food and drink for a period of time. It is practised all over the world for religious, cultural, or traditional reasons [1]. There are many different fasting methods. Perhaps the most well-known example of fasting is Ramadan. This intermittent fasting regime is carried out due to religious beliefs and involves not eating or drinking from sunrise to sunset for 30 consecutive days [1]. However, fasting is also used in the medical world. Since ancient Greece, it has been an established medical treatment and has been adopted into modern western medicine [1]. Recent research has identified many possible health benefits from fasting, and we now know more about the physiological effects of fasting than ever before.

Fasting throughout history
For centuries, our human ancestors did not have a three-course meal and were lucky if they had a single meal every day. As a result, the human body has evolved to cope with a scarcity of food. However, what evolution failed to factor in was our newfound ability to generate more food than is necessary. Therefore, the human body is not accustomed to the abundance of food available today and the rates at which it is consumed.

Consequently, the prevalence of obesity, and the associated health risks, is increasing. In 2015, obesity affected over 603 million adults worldwide, and its prevalence has increased continuously in most countries for the last 40 years [2]. Shockingly, obesity prevalence has doubled in more than 70 countries since 1980 [2]. Obesity is associated with many chronic diseases, including cardiovascular disease, diabetes, cancer, and musculoskeletal disorders [2]. Consequently, obesity accounted for four million deaths globally in 2015, with around two-thirds of these related to cardiovascular diseases [2]. These findings show the dangers of overeating food and, in turn, suggest that the reduction of food consumption through fasting may have many health benefits.

Types of fasting
There are four main types of fasting. They are
1. Water fast
2. Time-restricted feeding/eating
3. Calorie restriction
4. Dietary restriction

Water fast involves consuming only water and not consuming any other nutrients. In the Bible, Jesus water-fasted for 40 days prior to commencing his ministry (Matthew 4:1-2, Luke 4:1-2). Medically, this can be achieved. The longest record of a water fast is that of Angus Barbier I, who fasted continuously for 382 days and lost a total of 21 stone. This is recorded in the Guinness Book of World Records [3].

Time-restricted feeding involves eating only during certain periods of the day. In this method of fasting, calories don't need to be counted as long as food intake is restricted within certain periods. It may start with a ten-hour fasting period (or usually an overnight fast) with a 14-hour eating period. Slowly the fasting period needs to be increased, and the eating period needs to be decreased. Weight loss and health benefits are accrued when eating is restricted to 6 to 10 hours in a day. The Ramadan fast is a type of time-restricted feeding.

Calorie restriction. This involves limiting the number of calories eaten for a few days in a week. The popular 5:2 diet is a calorie-restricted diet and involves eating less than 500 calories for two days of the week.

Dietary restriction. This involves limiting the type of foods eaten during certain periods. The majority of the Christian fasting practised very commonly in the Orthodox Church involves dietary restriction. They practise dietary restriction for about 200 days every year. This is usually weekly on a Wednesday and a Friday. In addition, there are three prolonged periods of fasting during the year; 40 days prior to Good Friday (Lent), 40 days prior to Christmas (Advent) and 15 days in the first two weeks of August, prior to the bodily lifting up of Mother Mary into heaven (Assumption fast). During these periods, believers abstain from meat, dairy, fish and eggs.

The advantages of the Mediterranean diet may also arise from the fasting practised

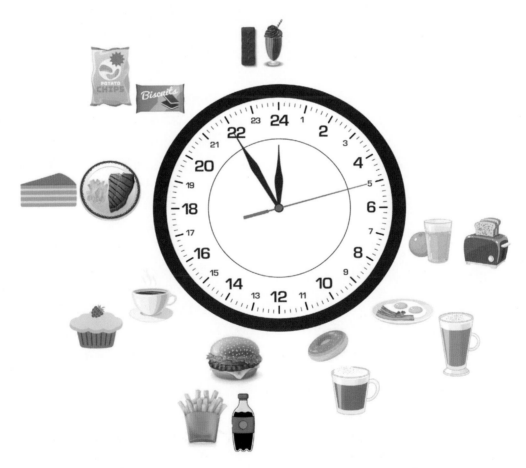

7 AM - Orange Juice & Toast
9 AM - Latte, Eggs & Bacon
11 AM - Doughnuts & Cappucino
1 PM - Burger, Drink & Chips
3:30 PM - Tea & Cakes

3:30 PM - Tea & Cakes
6:30 PM - Steak, Chips & Dessert
9 PM - Crisps & Biscuits while watching TV
12 Midnight - Midnight Chocolate Bar & Shake before bed

Snacking for 17 hours is unlikely to help in losing weight

Adventists also abstain from meats providing the good health seen in the Blue Zone areas like Loma Linda. The popular Keto diet is another type of dietary restriction where carbohydrates are restricted, and fats and proteins are consumed in excess. Unfortunately, there are some adverse reports regarding the Keto diet. Evidence shows that both low carbohydrate and high-carbohydrate diets are detrimental and increase mortality. Moderate amounts of carbohydrates provide the best diet and improve longevity.

Why fasting?

When we eat, the food consumed is broken down in the gut and is then absorbed. The main three components of food are carbohydrates, proteins and fat. Glucose produced following the breakdown of carbohydrates is the primary fuel source for most of the cells in our body. After a meal, excess glucose in the body cannot be used as fuel at that moment. This excess glucose is then stored up to be used between meals. There are potentially two different mechanisms by which this excess glucose is stored. The excess glucose is stored either as glycogen in the liver or as fat in the adipose tissue. There is, however, a finite limit to the amount of glycogen that can be stored in the liver. Usually, the glycogen stored in the liver can only last for about 12 to 24 hours before it is depleted. If a further meal is not eaten before that period, the body uses the stored fat.

Normally the fat is broken down into ketones, which can also be used as fuel by

different cells in the body. If required, the fat can also be converted back into glucose in the liver. Ideally, to lose weight, the body needs to enter prolonged periods of fasting (more than 10 to 12 hours) when the glycogen stores are used up, and the body starts utilising fuel from the fat stores. If meals are taken very frequently, the body only uses the glycogen stores between meals and, unfortunately, does not utilise the fat stores. Hence, constant feeding or snacking slowly builds up the body fat and does not allow the body fat to be used up for energy. Prolonged exercise can deplete the glycogen stores. However, if following or during the exercise, sugars are consumed, then the fat stores will not be accessed. The body will use the glucose from the consumed sugars as fuel in preference to the ketones from the fat stores. Nevertheless, when there is a prolonged period of fasting, then the body uses the fat stores after the glycogen stores have been exhausted. Hence any weight

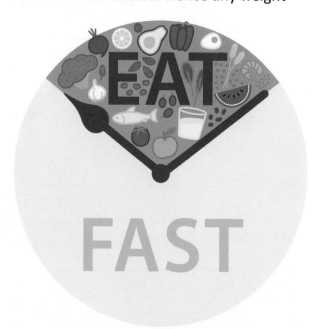

Eat for 8 hours and fast for 16 hours per day

reduction programme can only be successful if it is accompanied by an adequate period of fasting to allow the fat stores to be broken down as fuel.

In real life, however, the wrong advice is provided both to adults and children. We are told that snacking is essential. Children in school are encouraged to have a snack midmorning at 11:00 and a snack in the evening during the half-time break at football training. Research surveys have identified that instead of eating three meals a day, humans are now consuming six to nine meals per day. Coffee with biscuits at 7:00, cereals as breakfast at 9:00, coffee with doughnuts at 11:00, lunch at 13:00, tea and cakes at 15:30, dinner at 18:00, evening snack while watching TV at 21:00 and a milkshake with a chocolate bar at 23:00 and just before bed. In this regime, eight meals are consumed in a day. This regime only provides an eight-hour fast, which is inadequate to deplete the glycogen stores and utilise the fat stores for energy. With such a regime, the only result would be increased obesity and the complications that ensue from excess weight.

What are the benefits of fasting?

Arthritis

Fasting therapy can have benefits in the management of rheumatoid arthritis. One study by Muller and team included 53 patients with rheumatoid arthritis [1]. The study group consisting of 27 patients were on a seven-to ten-day sub-total fast followed by a vegan, gluten-free diet for three months. This was then followed by a lacto-vegetarian diet for a further nine months. The control group of 26 patients were allowed to eat an ordinary diet throughout the whole period. Even at the end of four weeks following the start of the study, the test group showed significant improvements in the number of tender and swollen joints, morning stiffness and grip strength. The benefits in the test group continued till the end of the study [1].

Fasting may also be beneficial in osteoarthritis [1]. One uncontrolled study asked 30 patients with osteoarthritis to follow an intermittent fasting regime for two weeks. The first three days were pre-fasting. During the following eight days, participants were provided with a calorie-restricted diet (300 calories) followed by a three-day re-feed program. There was significant improvement within the two weeks of the program. At the four-week and the twelve-week follow-up, significant pain relief, improved joint function and improvements in overall quality of life were still observed [1].

Cognitive functioning

Although little research has been done regarding intermittent fasting and cognitive function, there have been a few papers published that investigate the effects of calorie restriction. In one clinical trial, 50 normal-to-overweight elderly subjects were split into three groups. The first group was required to reduce their calorie intake by 30%, whilst the second was told to increase their intake of unsaturated fat by 20% [4]. The third group made no change to their diet. Memory performance was measured both at the onset of the study and three months later. The study found that patients who restricted their calories had an average 20% increase in verbal memory scores, a significant increase when compared to the other two groups [4].

A second study involved eighty obese participants, all aged over 60 years. Half of the participants were given specialist guidance on calorie restriction, whilst the other half received generic medical care – both for 12 months. The study found that participants who decreased their calorie intake and reduced their body mass index had significant improvements in verbal memory, verbal fluency, executive function, and global cognition [4].

In the modern-day world, food may be plentiful, but that was not the situation hundreds of years ago. Food was really scarce then. Members of a family or a group would not have any food for days. As stated previously, the metabolism would switch from using glucose as the fuel to using ketones as fuel. Surprisingly, mental acuity and response times are better when the brain is using ketones as fuel. This might have been an evolutionary adaptation that was gained for the survival of the species. A tiger hunts better when it is hungry. Similarly, a hungry hunter-gatherer had more skill and acumen to hunt or gather food.

Obesity

Obesity, which describes people who are massively overweight, is a huge health problem. It can cause many health issues, including an increased risk of cardiovascular disease and diabetes.

Additionally, 13 different cancers have been linked with obesity, including thyroid cancer, colon cancer and gallbladder cancer [5]. It is clear then that excessive weight is detrimental to health, and weight management is vital in maintaining well-being. Thankfully, fasting may be an effective intervention for obesity and weight loss. A review by Mattson and team analysed the available literature and found that studies involving alternate-day fasting reduced participants' weight by as much as 7% and decreased body fat by as much as 5.5 kilograms [5]. Even partaking in 5:2, intermittent fasting reduces a person's overall weekly calorie intake by 25% [5]. Such a reduction in calories will have a significant weight-loss effect, reducing the risk of the health problems associated with being obese or overweight.

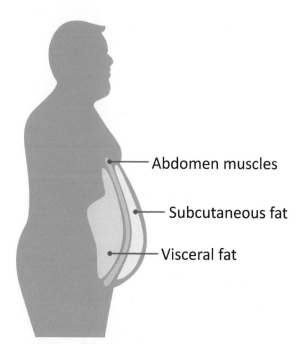

The body will only burn fat as fuel after the sugar stored in the liver is used up

Cancer

As previously stated, obesity is linked with certain types of cancer. The beneficial effects that fasting can have on weight are likely to reduce the risk of these cancers [4]. Not only this, but intermittent fasting is thought to impair the ability of cancerous cells to use energy, thereby reducing their growth and making them more responsive to treatments [3]. In addition, periodic fasting for two or more days can be as effective as chemotherapy in delaying the progression of a number of various cancers [4]. Fasting like this has also been shown to protect healthy cells from the toxic effects of chemotherapy whilst increasing the cancerous cells' sensitivity to the treatment [4].

Diabetes

Poor glucose metabolism may lead to the development of diabetes and is both a cause and consequence of the disease. When the body cannot metabolise glucose, blood sugars become elevated, and insulin resistance becomes greater. Insulin resistance is the driving factor in the development of diabetes. Fasting, by improving glucose metabolism, which increases insulin sensitivity, can therefore prevent the onset and progression of the disease. More recent studies have shown that intermittent fasting for three days a week reverses insulin resistance in patients with prediabetes and Type II diabetes [3]. Insulin resistance is the opposite of insulin sensitivity. Whilst reductions in insulin sensitivity have adverse effects, decreases in insulin resistance are beneficial. Fasting can therefore have a two-way beneficial effect on diabetes. Furthermore, the people of the Blue Zone Okinawa, who often follow an intermittent fasting regime and a calorie-restricted diet, have extremely low rates of obesity and diabetes, as well as significant longevity [3].

What can you do?

Break-FAST

Abstaining from food for 24 hours is a hard task and one that many people might not feel comfortable doing. Fortunately, benefits can be reaped by following the simplest form of fasting – "daily time-restricted feeding". As previously described, this type of fasting only allows people to eat during a certain timeframe within the day, reducing their opportunity to consume unnecessary calories. This can help with weight- management and will prevent the development of obesity. The fast can then be broken with a healthy morning meal. Make breakfast a true breaking of the fast. After breakfast, try eating your last meal within six hours. In total, during a 24-hour period, eat for six hours and then fast for 18 hours. Do this gradually over a period of time. If you are only used to fasting for ten hours, i.e., from 21:00 to 7:00, slowly increase this period over many weeks. 30 minutes per week could be a reasonable compromise. Start by eating the last meal of the day at 20:30 and breakfast the following morning at 7:00. In the following week, eat the last meal by 20:30 and eat breakfast the following morning at 7:30. Slowly decrease the time of eating to achieve an 18-hour fast and a 6-hour eating period. Please consult your doctor for further advice.

References

Chapter 1 – Blue Zones

1. Buettner D, Skemp S. Blue Zones: Lessons From the World's Longest Lived. Am J Lifestyle Med. 2016 Jul 7;10(5):318-321.
2. Mishra BN. Secret of eternal youth; teaching from the centenarian hot spots ("Blue Zones"). Indian J Community Med. 2009;34(4):273-275.
3. Mental health facts and statistics. Mind. [Online] April 2017. [Cited: February 19, 2021.]
4. Many mental illnesses reduce life expectancy more than heavy smoking. University of Oxford. [Online] May 23, 2014. [Cited: February 19, 2021.]
5. British Heart Foundation. CV STATISTICS – BHF UK FACTSHEET. British Heart Foundation. [Online] February 2018. [Cited: February 19, 2021.]
6. Laudicella M, Walsh B, Burns E, Smith PC. Cost of care for cancer patients in England: evidence from population-based patient-level data. Br J Cancer. 2016;114(11):1286- 1292.
7. Le LT, Sabaté J. Beyond meatless, the health effects of vegan diets: findings from the Adventist cohorts. Nutrients. 2014;6(6):2131-2147. Published 2014 May 27.

Chapter 2 – Avoid Sedentary Lifestyle - Age Healthily

1. Harvey JA, Chastin SF, Skelton DA. How Sedentary are Older People? A Systematic Review of the Amount of Sedentary Behavior. J Aging Phys Act. 2015;23(3):471-487.
2. Schrempft S, Jackowska M, Hamer M, Steptoe A. Associations between social isolation, loneliness, and objective physical activity in older men and women. BMC Public Health. 2019;19(1):74. Published 2019 Jan 16.
3. Booth FW, Roberts CK, Laye MJ. Lack of exercise is a major cause of chronic diseases. Compr Physiol. 2012;2(2):1143-1211.
4. Yan S, Fu W, Wang C, Mao J, Liu B, Zou L, Lv C. Association between sedentary behavior and the risk of dementia: a systematic review and meta-analysis. Transl Psychiatry. 2020 Apr 21;10(1):112.
5. Kim Y, Lee E. The association between elderly people's sedentary behaviors and their health-related quality of life: focusing on comparing the young-old and the old-old. Health Qual Life Outcomes 17, 131 (2019).
6. de Rezende LF, Rey-López JP, Matsudo VK, do Carmo Luiz O. Sedentary behavior and health outcomes among older adults: a systematic review. BMC Public Health. 2014 Apr 9.
7. Lugo D, Pulido AL, Mihos CG, Issa O, Cusnir M, Horvath SA, Lin J, Santana O. The effects of physical activity on cancer prevention, treatment and prognosis: A review of the literature. Complement Ther Med. 2019 Jun;44:9-13.
8. Fries JF, Bruce B, Chakravarty E. Compression of morbidity 1980-2011: a focused review of paradigms and progress. J Aging Res. 2011;2011:261702.
9. Chakravarty EF, Hubert HB, Lingala VB, Fries JF. Reduced disability and mortality among aging runners: a 21-year longitudinal study [published correction appears in Arch Intern Med. 2008 Dec 8;168(22):2496]. Arch Intern

Med. 2008;168(15):1638-1646.

10. NHS. Physical activity guidelines for older adults. NHS England. [Online] July 11, 2015. [Cited: February 08, 2018.]

Chapter 3 – Under-Standing Over-Sitting

1. Levine JA. Sick of sitting. Diabetologia. 2015;58(8):1751-1758.
2. Chau JY, Grunseit AC, Chey T, et al. Daily sitting time and all-cause mortality: a meta-analysis. PLoS One. 2013;8(11):e80000.
3. Veerman JL, Healy GN, Cobiac LJ, et al. Television viewing time and reduced life expectancy: a life table analysis [published correction appears in Br J Sports Med. 2012 Dec;46(16):1144]. Br J Sports Med. 2012;46(13):927-930.
4. Gómez-Cabello A, Vicente-Rodríguez G, Pindado M, et al. Mayor riesgo de obesidad y obesidad central en mujeres post-menopáusicas sedentarias [Increased risk of obesity and central obesity in sedentary postmenopausal women]. Nutr Hosp. 2012;27(3):865-870.
5. Vallance JK, Gardiner PA, Lynch BM, et al. Evaluating the Evidence on Sitting, Smoking, and Health: Is Sitting Really the New Smoking?. Am J Public Health. 2018;108(11):1478-1482.
6. Szczygieł E, Zielonka K, Mętel S, Golec J. Musculo-skeletal and pulmonary effects of sitting position - a systematic review. Ann Agric Environ Med. 2017;24(1):8-12.
7. Gupta N, Christiansen CS, Hallman DM, Korshøj M, Carneiro IG, Holtermann A. Is objectively measured sitting time associated with low back pain? A cross-sectional investigation in the NOMAD study. PLoS One. 2015;10(3):e0121159.

8. Nachemson A. The load on lumbar disks in different positions of the body. Clin Orthop Relat Res. 1966;45:107-122.
9. Keegan JJ. Alterations of the lumbar curve related to posture and seating. J Bone Joint Surg Am. 1953;35-A(3):589-603.
10. De Geer CM. Intervertebral Disk Nutrients and Transport Mechanisms in Relation to Disk Degeneration: A Narrative Literature Review. J Chiropr Med. 2018;17(2):97-105.

Chapter 4 – Television and Its Effects on Brain Function

1. Zayed, Y. (2021). TV licence fee statistics. House of Commons Library Briefing Paper no. CBP-8101. London: House of Commons Library. [Online] [Accessed on 8th July 2021]. https://researchbriefings.files.parliament.uk/documents/CBP-8101/CBP-8101.pdf
2. Depp CA, Schkade DA, Thompson WK, Jeste DV. Age, affective experience, and television use. Am J Prev Med. 2010;39(2):173-178.
3. Fancourt D, Steptoe A. Television viewing and cognitive decline in older age: findings from the English Longitudinal Study of Ageing. Sci Rep. 2019;9(1):2851
4. Hoang TD, Reis J, Zhu N, et al. Effect of Early Adult Patterns of Physical Activity and Television Viewing on Midlife Cognitive Function. JAMA Psychiatry. 2016;73(1):73-79.
5. Grace MS, Dillon F, Barr ELM, Keadle SK, Owen N, Dunstan DW. Television Viewing Time and Inflammatory-Related Mortality. Med Sci Sports Exerc. 2017;49(10):2040-2047.
6. Suzuki K. Chronic Inflammation as an

Immunological Abnormality and Effectiveness of Exercise. Biomolecules. 2019;9(6):223.

Chapter 5 – What Is Arthritis?

1. Ngian G.S. Rheumatoid arthritis. Aust Fam Physician. 2010 Sep;39(9):626-8.
2. Richmond SA, Fukuchi RK, Ezzat A, Schneider K, Schneider G, Emery CA. Are joint injury, sport activity, physical activity, obesity, or occupational activities predictors for osteoarthritis? A systematic review. J Orthop Sports Phys Ther. 2013 Aug;43(8):515-B19.
3. Culliford DJ, Maskell J, Kiran A, et al. The lifetime risk of total hip and knee arthroplasty: results from the UK general practice research database. Osteoarthr Cartil. 2012;20(6):519–24.
4. National Joint Registry. NJR 17th Annual Report 2020. National Joint Registry [Online] 2020. [Cited October 2020]
5. Halawi MJ, Jongbloed W, Baron S, Savoy L, Williams VJ, Cote MP. Patient Dissatisfaction After Primary Total Joint Arthroplasty: The Patient Perspective. J Arthroplasty. 2019;34(6):1093-1096.
6. Gunaratne R, Pratt DN, Banda J, Fick DP, Khan RJK, Robertson BW. Patient Dissatisfaction Following Total Knee Arthroplasty: A Systematic Review of the Literature. J Arthroplasty. 2017;32(12):3854- 3860.
7. Choosing Wisely UK About Choosing Wisely UK Choosing Wisely UK [Online] 2020. [Cited October 2020]
8. Järvinen TL, Sihvonen R, Englund M. Arthroscopy for degenerative knee--a difficult habit to break?. Acta Orthop. 2014;85(3):215-217.
9. Rongen JJ, Rovers MM, van Tienen TG, Buma P, Hannink G. Increased risk for knee replacement surgery after arthroscopic surgery for degenerative meniscal tears: a multi-center longitudinal observational study using data from the osteoarthritis initiative. Osteoarthritis Cartilage. 2017 Jan;25(1):23-29.
10. Charlesworth J, Fitzpatrick J, Perera NKP, Orchard J. Osteoarthritis- a systematic review of long-term safety implications for osteoarthritis of the knee. BMC Musculoskelet Disord. 2019;20(1):151. Published 2019 Apr 9.

Chapter 6 – Red Meat

1. Wolk A. Potential health hazards of eating red meat. J Intern Med. 2017;281(2):106-122.
2. Bouvard V, Loomis D, Guyton KZ et al. Carcinogenicity of consumption of red and processed meat. Lancet Oncol 2015; 16: 1599–600.
3. Feskens EJ, Sluik D, van Woudenbergh GJ. Meat consumption, diabetes, and its complications. Curr Diab Rep. 2013;13(2):298-306.
4. Haring B, Misialek JR, Rebholz CM, et al. Association of Dietary Protein Consumption With Incident Silent Cerebral Infarcts and Stroke: The Atherosclerosis Risk in Communities (ARIC) Study. Stroke. 2015;46(12):3443-3450.
5. Bernstein AM, Sun Q, Hu FB, Stampfer MJ, Manson JE, Willett WC. Major dietary protein sources and risk of coronary heart disease in women. Circulation. 2010;122(9):876-883.
6. Kaluza J, Åkesson A, Wolk A. Long-term processed and unprocessed red meat consumption and risk of heart failure: A prospective cohort study of women. Int J Cardiol. 2015;193:42-46.

7. Larsson SC, Orsini N. Red meat and processed meat consumption and all-cause mortality: a meta-analysis. Am J Epidemiol. 2014;179(3):282-289.

Chapter 7 – Dairy

1. Silanikove N, Leitner G, Merin U. The Interrelationships between Lactose Intolerance and the Modern Dairy Industry: Global Perspectives in Evolutional and Historical Backgrounds. Nutrients. 2015;7(9):7312-7331.

2. FAO. Gateway to Dairy Production and Products. 2018. FAO. Food and Agriculture Organization of the United Nations.

3. Weaver CM, Proulx WR, Heaney R. Choices for achieving adequate dietary calcium with a vegetarian diet. Am J Clin Nutr. 1999;70(3 Suppl):543S-548S.

4. Bian S, Hu J, Zhang K, Wang Y, Yu M, Ma J. Dairy product consumption and risk of hip fracture: a systematic review and meta-analysis. BMC Public Health. 2018;18(1):165. Published 2018 Jan 22.

5. Song Y, Chavarro JE, Cao Y, et al. Whole milk intake is associated with prostate cancer-specific mortality among U.S. male physicians. J Nutr. 2013;143:189-196.

6. Chan JM, Stampfer MJ, Giovannucci E, et al. Plasma insulin-like growth factor-1 and prostate cancer risk: a prospective study. Science. 1998;279:563–565.

7. Giovannucci E. Insulin, insulin-like growth factors and colon cancer: a review of the evidence. J Nutr. 2001;131(11 Suppl):3109S-20S.

8. Fraser GE, Jaceldo-Siegl K, Orlich M, Mashchak A, Sirirat R, Knutsen S. Dairy, soy, and risk of breast cancer: those confounded milks. Int J Epidemiol. 2020;49(5):1526-1537.

9. Kushi LH, Mink PJ, Folsom AR, et al. Prospective study of diet and ovarian cancer. Am J Epidemiol. 1999;149:21–31.

10. Section on Breastfeeding. Breastfeeding and the use of human milk. Pediatrics. 2012;129(3):e827-e841.

Chapter 8 – Food from Plants

1. Orlich MJ, Singh PN, Sabaté J, et al. Vegetarian dietary patterns and mortality in Adventist Health Study 2. JAMA Intern Med. 2013;173(13):1230-1238.

2. Clinton CM, O'Brien S, Law J, Renier CM, Wendt MR. Whole-foods, plant-based diet alleviates the symptoms of osteoarthritis. Arthritis. 2015;2015:708152.

3. McDougall J., Bruce B., Spiller G., Westerdahl J., McDougall M. Effects of a very low-fat, vegan diet in subjects with rheumatoid arthritis. The Journal of Alternative and Complementary Medicine. 2002;8(1):71–75.

4. Barnard ND, Goldman DM, Loomis JF, et al. Plant-Based Diets for Cardiovascular Safety and Performance in Endurance Sports. Nutrients. 2019;11(1):130. Published 2019 Jan 10.

5. Kahleova H, Levin S, Barnard N. Cardio-Metabolic Benefits of Plant-Based Diets. Nutrients. 2017;9(8):848. Published 2017 Aug 9.

6. NHS Digital. Statistics on Obesity, Physical Activity and Diet, England 2020. NHS Digital. [Online] 2020. [Cited October 2020].

7. de Gavelle E, Huneau JF, Bianchi CM, Verger EO, Mariotti F. Protein Adequacy Is Primarily a Matter of

Protein Quantity, Not Quality: Modeling an Increase in Plant :Animal Protein Ratio in French Adults. Nutrients. 2017 Dec 8;9(12).

8. Li C, Fang A, Ma W et al. Amount Rather than Animal vs Plant Protein Intake Is Associated with Skeletal Muscle Mass in Community-Dwelling Middle-Aged and Older Chinese Adults: Results from the Guangzhou Nutrition and Health Study. J Acad Nutr Diet. 2019 Sep;119(9):1501-1510.

Chapter 9 – Natural Alternatives to Medicine

1. Jiang TA. Health Benefits of Culinary Herbs and Spices. J AOAC Int. 2019;102(2):395-411.
2. Wu MS, Aquino LBB, Barbaza MYU, et al. Anti-Inflammatory and Anticancer Properties of Bioactive Compounds from Sesamum indicum L.-A Review. Molecules. 2019;24(24):4426.
3. Maćkowiak K, Torlińska-Walkowiak N, Torlińska B. Dietary fibre as an important constituent of the diet. Postepy Hig Med Dosw (Online). 2016;70:104-109. Published 2016 Feb 25.
4. Rusu ME, Mocan A, Ferreira ICFR, Popa DS. Health Benefits of Nut Consumption in Middle-Aged and Elderly Population. Antioxidants (Basel). 2019;8(8):302. Published 2019
5. Meng X, Li Y, Li S, et al. Dietary Sources and Bioactivities of Melatonin. Nutrients. 2017;9(4):367. Published 2017 Apr 7.
6. Messina V. Nutritional and health benefits of dried beans. Am J Clin Nutr. 2014 Jul;100 Suppl 1:437S-42S.

Chapter 10 – The Microbiome (Gut Bacteria)

1. Cresci GA, Bawden E. Gut Microbiome: What We Do and Don't Know. Nutr Clin Pract. 2015;30(6):734-746.
2. Nagpal R, Mainali R, Ahmadi S, et al. Gut microbiome and aging: Physiological and mechanistic insights. Nutr Healthy Aging. 2018;4(4):267-285. Published 2018 Jun 15.
3. Lorenzo D, GianVincenzo Z, Carlo Luca R, Karan G, Jorge V, Roberto M, Javad P. Oral- Gut Microbiota and Arthritis: Is There an Evidence-Based Axis? J Clin Med. 2019 Oct 22;8(10):0.
4. Kho ZY, Lal SK. The Human Gut Microbiome - A Potential Controller of Wellness and Disease. Front Microbiol. 2018;9:1835. Published 2018 Aug 14.
5. David LA, Maurice CF, Carmody RN, et al. Diet rapidly and reproducibly alters the human gut microbiome. Nature. 2014 Jan 23;505(7484):559-63.
6. Rezac S, Kok CR, Heermann M, Hutkins R. Fermented Foods as a Dietary Source of Live Organisms. Front Microbiol. 2018;9:1785. Published 2018 Aug 24.
7. Markowiak P, Śliżewska K. Effects of Probiotics, Prebiotics, and Synbiotics on Human Health. Nutrients. 2017 Sep 15;9(9):1021.

Chapter 11 – Rest and Relaxation

1. Medic G, Wille M, Hemels ME. Short- and long-term health consequences of sleep disruption. Nat Sci Sleep. 2017;9:151-161. Published 2017 May 19.
2. Kim TW, Jeong JH, Hong SC. The impact of sleep and circadian disturbance on hormones and metabolism. Int J Endocrinol. 2015;2015:591729.
3. Tononi G, Cirelli C. Sleep function and

synaptic homeostasis. Sleep Med Rev. 2006;10:49-62.

4. Nédélec M, Halson S, Abaidia AE, Ahmaidi S, Dupont G. Stress, Sleep and Recovery in Elite Soccer: A Critical Review of the Literature. Sports Med. 2015;45(10):1387- 1400.

5. Shechter A, Kim EW, St-Onge MP, Westwood AJ. Blocking nocturnal blue light for insomnia: A randomized controlled trial. J Psychiatr Res. 2018;96:196-202.

6. Guimaraes LH, de Carvalho LB, Yanaguibashi G, do Prado GF. Physically active elderly women sleep more and better than sedentary women. Sleep Medicine. 2008 Jul 1;9(5):488-93.

7. Sauder KA, McCrea CE, Ulbrecht JS, Kris- Etherton PM, West SG. Pistachio nut consumption modifies systemic hemodynamics, increases heart rate variability, and reduces ambulatory blood pressure in well-controlled type 2 diabetes: a randomized trial. J Am Heart Assoc. 2014;3(4).

Chapter 12 – Family and Friends

1. Aesop. (1999). The Lion and the Mouse. In C.E. Tiger (Ed.), The Classic Treasury of Aesops Fables (pp. 47). Pennsylvania: Running Press Book Publishers.

2. Sharma R. The Family and Family Structure Classification Redefined for the Current Times. J Family Med Prim Care. 2013;2(4):306-310.

3. Thomas PA, Liu H, Umberson D. Family Relationships and Well-Being. Innov Aging. 2017;1(3):igx025.

4. Holt-Lunstad J, Smith TB, Layton JB. Social relationships and mortality risk: a

meta- analytic review. PLoS Med. 2010;7(7):e1000316. Published 2010 Jul 27.

5. Brent LJ, Chang SW, Gariépy JF, Platt ML. The neuroethology of friendship. Ann N Y Acad Sci. 2014;1316(1):1-17.

6. Shensa A, Sidani JE, Dew MA, Escobar-Viera CG, Primack BA. Social Media Use and Depression and Anxiety Symptoms: A Cluster Analysis. Am J Health Behav.2018;42(2):116-128.

7. Modig K, Talbäck M, Torssander J, Ahlbom A. Payback time? Influence of having children on mortality in old age. J Epidemiol Community Health. 2017;71(5):424-430.

8. Barclay K, Kolk M. Parity and Mortality: An Examination of Different Explanatory Mechanisms Using Data on Biological and Adoptive Parents. Eur J Popul. 2018;35(1):63-85. Published 2018 Feb 21. doi:10.1007/s10680-018-9469-1.

9. Buettner D, Skemp S. Blue Zones: Lessons From the World's Longest Lived. Am J Lifestyle Med. 2016;10(5):318-321. Published 2016 Jul 7.

Chapter 13 – Ikigai – Japanese for "Purpose in Life"

1. Musich S, Wang SS, Kraemer S, Hawkins K, Wicker E. Purpose in Life and Positive Health Outcomes Among Older Adults. Popul Health Manag. 2018;21(2):139-147.

2. Sone T, Nakaya N, Ohmori K, et al. Sense of life worth living (ikigai) and mortality in Japan: Ohsaki Study. Psychosom Med. 2008;70(6):709-715.

3. Buettner D. The Blue Zones. Washington, D.C.: National Geographic

Society; 2010.

4. Boyle PA, Buchman AS, Barnes LL, Bennett DA. Effect of a purpose in life on risk of incident Alzheimer disease and mild cognitive impairment in community-dwelling older persons. Arch Gen Psychiatry. 2010;67(3):304-310.

5. Hill PL, Turiano NA. Purpose in life as a predictor of mortality across adulthood. Psychol Sci. 2014;25(7):1482- 1486.

Chapter 14 – Faith

1. WIN-Gallup International. Global Index of Religiousity and Atheism; 2012. [Cited October 2020].

2. Hill TD, Ellison CG, Burdette AM, Taylor J, Friedman KL. Dimensions of religious involvement and leukocyte telomere length. Soc Sci Med. 2016 Aug;163:168-75. Epub 2016 Apr 28. PMID: 27174242.

3. Agli O, Bailly N, Ferrand C. Spirituality and religion in older adults with dementia: a systematic review. Int Psychogeriatr. 2015 May;27(5):715-25.

4. Banerjee, A.T., Boyle, M.H., Anand, S.S. et al. The Relationship Between Religious Service Attendance and Coronary Heart Disease and Related Risk Factors in Saskatchewan, Canada. J Relig Health 53, 141–156 (2014).

5. Jim HS, Pustejovsky JE, Park CL, Danhauer SC, Sherman AC, Fitchett G, Merluzzi TV, Munoz AR, George L, Snyder MA, Salsman JM. Religion, spirituality, and physical health in cancer patients: A meta-analysis. Cancer. 2015 Nov 1;121(21):3760-8.

6. Baetz M, Bowen R. Chronic pain and fatigue: Associations with religion and spirituality. Pain Res Manag. 2008 Sep-Oct;13(5):383-8.

7. Snell S, Hughes T, Fore C, Lukman R,

Morgan B. Treating Chronic Nonmalignant Pain: Evidence and Faith-Based Approaches. J Christ Nurs. 2019 Jan/Mar;36(1):22-30.

Chapter 15 – Fasting

1. Michalsen A, Li C. Fasting therapy for treating and preventing disease - current state of evidence. Forsch Komplementmed. 2013;20(6):444-453.

2. GBD 2015 Obesity Collaborators, Afshin A, Forouzanfar MH, et al. Health Effects of Overweight and Obesity in 195 Countries over 25 Years. N Engl J Med. 2017;377(1):13- 27.

3. Stewart WK, Fleming LW. Features of a successful therapeutic fast of 382 days' duration. Postgrad Med J. 1973;49(569):203-209.

4. de Cabo R, Mattson MP. Effects of Intermittent Fasting on Health, Aging, and Disease. N Engl J Med. 2019 Dec 26;381(26):2541-2551

5. Mattson MP, Longo VD, Harvie M. Impact of intermittent fasting on health and disease processes. Ageing Res Rev. 2017;39:46-58.

Printed in Great Britain
by Amazon